"The patient engagement is key to better patient outcomes, lower costs of care, and more joyful clinicians. Health care needs people like Brian Boyle to keep us focused on the goal, to have an impact."
—Dr. Peter Pronovost, Johns Hopkins Medicine

THE PATIENT EXPERIENCE

THE PATIENT EXPERIENCE

The Importance of Care, Communication, and Compassion in the Hospital Room

BRIAN BOYLE

Skyhorse Publishing

Skyhorse Publishing books may be purchased in bulk at special discounts for sales promotion, corporate gifts, fund-raising, or educational purposes. Special editions can also be created to specifications. For details, contact the Special Sales Department, Skyhorse Publishing, 307 West 36th Street, 11th Floor, New York, NY 10018 or info@skyhorsepublishing.com.

Skyhorse® and Skyhorse Publishing® are registered trademarks of Skyhorse Publishing, Inc.®, a Delaware corporation.

Visit our website at www.skyhorsepublishing.com.

10 9 8 7 6 5 4 3 2 1

Library of Congress Cataloging-in-Publication Data is available on file.

Cover design: David Ter-Avanesyan
Cover images: Shutterstock

Hardcover ISBN: 978-1-63220-710-4
Paperback ISBN: 978-1-5107-7371-4
Ebook ISBN: 978-1-63220-929-0

Printed in the United States of America

In my moment of pain,
You gave me comfort.

In my vision of darkness,
You gave me light.

In my world of loneliness,
You held my hand.

In my hour of doubt,
You gave me hope.

In my time of dying,
You gave me life.

This book is dedicated to all the individuals who have chosen to pursue their life's work in health care. Thank you for choosing this path and for all the good that you do.

CONTENTS

FOREWORD

"*A*LTHOUGH THE WORLD IS FULL OF SUFFERING, IT IS ALSO FULL OF THE
OVERCOMING OF IT.*" —Helen Keller*

IT IS ODD TO THINK THAT THE CIRCUMSTANCES THAT BROUGHT BRIAN
Boyle into our lives are ones we would not wish on our worst enemies.
Yet, we are eternally grateful for knowing him and his family, and our
lives will forever be enriched by our shared experiences.

In 2004, Brian was in a horrific car crash that left him clinging to life
in a hospital bed. The months of agony he endured during recovery and
the triumph of his incredible spirit over adversity are chronicled in his
2009 book, *Iron Heart.*

After the crash, Brian and his parents, JoAnn and Garth, found
themselves thrust into a scary and lonely environment in which they had
little control. At the darkest time in their lives, they placed their hope
and faith in the women and men who chose as their life's work to heal
the sick. Those strangers soon became friends and later, a second family.

We met Brian in 2010 and, as educators, we encouraged him to share his
experiences and what he had learned firsthand as a patient near death—in

a medically induced coma—with the hope of changing health care for the better. Perhaps the greatest lesson the Boyle family learned and later shared is that the miracles he achieved were not solitary accomplishments. In this book, Brian likens the effort to that of a relay team, where each member has an essential part to play for the team to be successful.

It is our sincere hope that families will recognize the important lessons in this story as they travel their own paths and understand the important role they play in the health of their loved ones, as well as their right and duty to be involved in their loved ones' care. As individuals who have spent many years working in the health care system and continue to do so, we also wish, for our colleagues, that they will approach this book with an open mind and heart and recognize that embracing the family as part of total patient care brings us closer to our reason for choosing this profession in the first place: to cure and care for those who need our help.

Brian and his family tell an incredibly raw story of survival and success, made possible only with the help of inspirational health care professionals. We can all learn from them.

Alison Burrows, MBA, RN, and Mark Rulle, EdD
The Maryland Healthcare Education Institute

PROLOGUE

THE WORLD IS FULL OF UNKNOWNS. WE WERE A NORMAL FAMILY LIVING a happy life, and then one day, a near-fatal car accident changed everything. The life we knew was shattered. For the next few months, we were constantly faced with unfathomable uncertainty and total despair.

While in a two-month-long medically induced coma, I was unable to move or talk to anyone around me, yet I was able to hear, see, and feel pain for a majority of my time in the Intensive Care Unit. As a family, we never thought that we would face such a traumatic situation, such a horrific nightmare. We were thrown into a place consisting of surgeries, machines, tubes, blood, and medical terms that caused utter confusion. We were in the hands of my medical team, and a few of them even said I was "in God's hands."

Life seems to go on standby when you enter this unfamiliar realm. You frequently come face to face with the strength of the human spirit and the perseverance of the mind and the body. Throughout this entire ordeal, my parents and I experienced how unforgiving life can be and how it can drastically change in the blink of an eye. There was no guidebook or support group to prepare us for what we were in for as a family.

What I learned throughout my time in the hospital is that while I may have been the patient lying in the hospital bed, I was not the only one in that room who was suffering. The observations that I made truly inspired me and helped me understand how important the role of communication is among the patient, family, and health care provider. When I was able to learn how to talk again, I soon discovered that the power of the voice is amplified when the message is of gratitude, that a simple smile cannot be underestimated, and that body language and tone of voice are critical components within the hospital room.

The idea of this book came about through many conversations with care providers all over the country. I always offer a question-and-answer session at the end of my health care presentations, and a question that is asked every single time is: What can care providers do better when it comes to treating the patient? In all honesty, I had trouble answering this question during my first few years of speaking about my experience. When they asked me this question, I explained that I am alive, breathing on my own, living life to the fullest, and I have my amazing care team to thank for that. I am also very positive and I rarely reflect on negative scenarios or experiences, but that answer did not satisfy them. They urged me to offer a few personal suggestions that I thought could help improve the patient experience, the quality of care, the communication, and the healing collaboration between patient and care provider.

When my parents attended my events with me, they were asked how care providers can improve the experience for the family in the hospital setting. After a lot of soul-searching, my parents and I came to the conclusion that our experiences not only could help other patients and families going through a similar ordeal, but also could help care providers offer the best possible care to those patients and families.

Every patient in the hospital has a story, and along with their loved ones, they share an experience. After all we have been through, we made the decision to put our thoughts and experiences together to share our sincere gratitude and insight with the medical community from a patient and family perspective. We also hope that our experiences can offer hope and guidance for families facing the heartbreaking sadness when an unexpected, life-altering medical situation occurs.

Throughout this book, my parents and I discuss what worked for us during our time in the hospital, along with some things that could have been done a little bit differently to improve the situation. In no way are we trying to declare that this is the only way to treat the patient because that is not our intention or place to say such things. Our goal is to offer suggestions that we hope will improve the overall experience for you, the patient, and his or her family.

This book is divided into five parts that deal with themes related to navigating the health care system:

- introduction of Brian's story and background
- topics that are related to caring for the patient
- the motivational impact of communication in the hospital room
- having compassion for the wants and needs of the patient and his or her family
- an overview of the information that is discussed in the book with a variety of exercises to help retain the material and apply it to your health care career

Each chapter begins with the following: the personal experiences of me and my parents in the hospital, with a strong emphasis on learning lessons that are supported by research; suggestions that we have made from those experiences; and a series of introspective, reflective questions for the care provider, which will also be included in the workbook exercises at the end of the book, where the provider will have a chance to write down answers.

Most of my recovery was spent in the ICU, but I strongly believe that the information we cover in this book can be very effective in any area of the hospital, as well as the entire health care system, because the end goal is taking better care of people. In order for us to provide better care for these individuals, we must understand the experiences they go through within the health care system. We must observe what they think and feel as they go through their journey. Our story is only one journey, and it is intended as a means to initiate the much-needed conversation of how we can take a step further to improve the experience for the patient and his or her family.

Whether you are a student who is planning on entering the health care field, a health care professional working indirectly with the patient, a veteran care provider with decades of frontline experience, a patient in the hospital, or a family that is currently going through the recovery process, this book provides a lot of valuable insight into the journey of healing that takes place within the hospital. The goal of this insight is to improve care, communication, and compassion in the hospital room.

Now let us take that next step forward and begin this journey of seeing life through the eyes of the patient. This is the patient experience.

PART ONE

FROM TRAGEDY TO TRIUMPH

"You don't know how strong you are until being strong is
the only choice you have."

—Anonymous

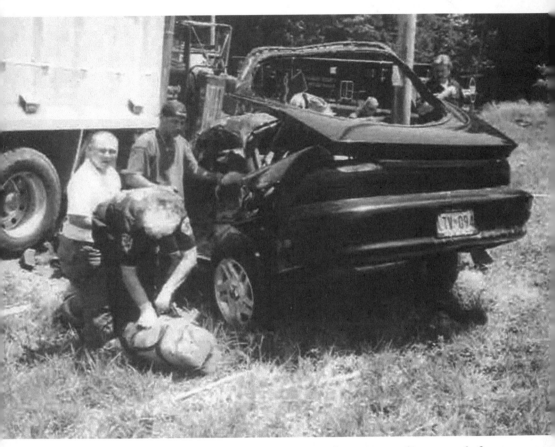

The accident scene on July 6, 2004. My EMS providers are attending to me before I am extricated from the vehicle and flown out by a medevac helicopter.

CHAPTER 1

JULY 6, 2004

*T*HE *PATIENT EXPERIENCE* BEGINS ONE MONTH AFTER I GRADUATED from high school in 2004. I was driving home from swim practice and was involved in a near-fatal car accident with a dump truck. The injuries were catastrophic: heart ripped across my chest; shattered ribs, clavicle, and pelvis; collapsed lungs; failure of the kidneys and laceration of the liver; concussion; 60 percent blood loss.

I was trapped in my car at the accident scene, and my EMS providers used the Jaws of Life to get me out of the vehicle in just enough time to be medevaced out. I had only fifteen minutes left to live, so time definitely was of the essence that day.

When I arrived at shock trauma, the main concern was my heart and safely getting the blood to stop flowing into places where it was not supposed to be going. My life was hanging by a delicate thread.

After several lifesaving operations, there was not much else for my loved ones to do but wait for over two months while I remained in a coma. I was told later that I was the worst patient in the unit for many weeks besides those who were on their way to the morgue. I had to be resuscitated eight times throughout the entire ordeal, so it was considered a monumental triumph just to be kept alive with the help of machines. Another day still on this Earth meant another victory, and so it went.

As far as the future, it did not exist. The chances of me leaving the hospital were possible, but only if I was transferred to a long-term nursing home. If, by chance, I did recover from the coma, walking was unthinkable due to my shattered pelvis. The thought of swimming was just that, only a thought. Like my body, my dreams were shattered.

In a chemically induced coma, I lay on my back paralyzed and in a state of total confusion. I woke up not knowing how I arrived there or what happened to me. Drugs that were many times stronger than morphine were flowing through my veins, and the life-support machines kept my lungs breathing and my heart beating.

My parents were suffering too. They watched over me every day as I struggled to stay alive. They are not medical people, so the terms and procedures were quite overwhelming to them. Approval signatures for surgeries were common at this point. They may not have fully understood the complicated procedures and did not have any medical records to review, but they believed in the entire medical team. They did learn a lot when they visited me, because the doctors and nurses would explain some of what was done in detail.

After spending two months in a coma, undergoing fourteen major operations, and receiving thirty-six blood transfusions and thirteen plasma treatments, I started to slowly regain consciousness. Each moment was a conscious effort to claw my way back to the living—a scary process, since my eyes were open, but I was paralyzed all over. Aware of my surroundings, I did my best to continue through the darkness. I chose to escape my mental prison and live life stronger. The other option was death.

A few weeks went by and progress was slow, from regaining the strength to smile, blink, move my fingers, wiggle my toes, and chew and swallow ice, to the point where I learned to talk again with the help of a speaking valve placed on my tracheostomy tube. When I regained my ability to talk, my life would be forever changed.

I lost a total of one hundred pounds while I was in the ICU, and then I was transferred to a rehab center in Baltimore where the healing slowly continued. The day after we arrived, my parents and I wanted to get some fresh air and tour the grounds. As they were pushing me along in my wheelchair, we were casually talking about the type of sessions that I had scheduled that day. We started to navigate down a small path along the side of the main building, and I soon realized that this was a part of the center that cared for the patients who were long term. A majority of these patients were in a vegetative state, and, unfortunately, quite a few of them would never come out of deep comas.

As we walked along these windows, I saw my reflection and a sense of dread instantly filled my mind because I realized there was a very good possibility that I could have just as easily been in that part of the hospital. My heart went out to these men and women, young and old.

Those patients were on my mind throughout the rest of that day, added onto the fact that I was also trying to mentally absorb everything that had taken place over the past two months. Even as I put on a happy face for the outside world, I had a lot of existential thoughts going through my mind, which were further intensified after seeing the patients in long-term care. I still had so many questions. I needed so many answers.

My health was improving, but was this progress only a false hope, the calm before the storm? Would I survive the night and live to see another day, another week? Would I make a full recovery, and if I did, what exactly is a full recovery for a person with my type of extensive injuries? Why did I have to go through all this? Why do bad things happen to good people? Why do we ask questions like this and rarely ever receive any answers? Would life ever be back to normal again? My mind started to get overwhelmed thinking about all the what-if possibilities and scenarios.

In the book titled *Everything Happens for a Reason*, Mira Kirshenbaum writes: "Once you find a personally compelling answer to the question, 'Why did this happen to me?' for the first time your attention is taken off the past that you cannot control and focused on your future, which you have some control over." With this in mind, one can try to accept what has happened in the past and start to realize the power one has in shaping the future.

I broke into a cold sweat just trying to imagine it, but this philosophical shock to the system started to evolve slowly into a different outlook on life. I started to realize that this whole ordeal was much more than dealing with the injuries sustained from a collision between two vehicles; it was dealing with life and the unforeseen obstacles we face every day. Confronting the negativity, interacting with the unexpected, and doing our best to overcome adversity.

Nobody really knows what tomorrow will bring. Even after all that I had gone through over the previous two months, I still did not have the slightest clue of what was going to happen next. I could only wonder and hope that it would be positive. That afternoon would end up making a profound impact on my life.

I was participating in my second physical therapy session, and my therapist recommended that I take a moment to rest. I began looking around at the other patients in the unit and reflecting on the journey back to life I took with my family. I thought about the extent and serious nature of my injuries, and the reality of having to spend the next few years recovering. I looked back on the experiences that I had in the hospital—the operations that kept me alive, the blood donations that kept life running through my veins, and the health care team that brought me back to life. I thought about the love from my family and friends, and the support that I received from people I had never met who were praying for me.

The tiny hairs rose on the back of my neck and my pulse quickened. Thoughts raced through my mind—about life, death, and why things are the way they are. My friends and loved ones looked at me as a living miracle, but I considered myself just a regular young guy who had been trying to get better each day. I was alive and I was grateful, but there was something else too.

I knew that the next few months and possibly years would be full of hardship and overcoming obstacles, but what brought me hope is that I could live to see those next few months and years. I may have been in a wheelchair and a hundred pounds lighter than I was before the accident, but I was no longer being kept alive with machines. I was not breathing with the aid of the ventilator, or being hooked up to the kidney dialysis machine or the other dozen medical devices that allowed blood and electricity to flow through my veins. My new life was just beginning.

Similar to the other injured patients in the unit, in the hospital, and throughout the world, I was clinging to life with a white-knuckled grip and I would never let go. I started to understand that I was more than just a teenage kid who was in a bad car accident and trying to live life stronger than death. To the people around me, I was a symbol of hope—a visual reminder that modern medicine combined with state-of-the-art technology, prayer, and the love of a family can help save a person's life.

Up until that moment in my wheelchair, my entire outlook was directed inward. I was asking personally reflective questions about why I was in a car accident, but in the long run, it was not about me at all.

I was asking the wrong questions because I was looking inward. I had to think about all the people who had helped me and the gift they had given me. I was alive, but the true gift they gave me was more than just existing; it was the ability to understand the hardships and tragedies that other people were going through and to be able to relate to them, to help them. It was a form of survivorship, an instant connection generated when you meet somebody who has been in or is currently going through a similar adverse situation. The experience is similar to the feeling you have when you are in a different part of the world and you find out the person you are talking to is from your hometown. It is a feeling of being intimately connected, but multiplied by a thousand.

The moment I started to regain full consciousness in the ICU, I became intensely focused on communicating with everyone around me—thanking them for all their hard work, reassuring everyone that I would be okay, and trying my best to show a positive attitude. However, it was not until that afternoon that I really started to confront the kind of future that I would have.

I do not know if everything happens for a reason, but I do know that I was meant to have this quiet reflection during that afternoon in my wheelchair. Even though I did not know why the accident happened to me, I now understood why I was saved.

I made a promise to myself in that wheelchair: if, when, I ever made a full recovery, I would dedicate my life to making a positive impact on the lives of the people around me. I would start out by personally thanking each and every one of the people who contributed to my survival—from the EMS providers at the accident scene to all my care providers in the hospital. I would become an advocate for blood donation and volunteer my time for the American Red Cross. I would meet and connect with other people who had undergone or were going through a similar bout of adversity. I would do all I could to speak on behalf of health care and become a patient advocate so that I could recommend various methods that I thought might improve the patient experience in the hospital.

I had a new outlook on life, and I was now on a mission. Throughout the rest of my physical therapy session, I interacted with the other patients in the room similar to the way that they interacted with me when I first arrived at rehab. Before I was wheeled into the unit, I was a complete stranger, but the moment I interacted with the other patients, I became a fellow survivor—and a friend.

Whatever their background, age, and type of injury or illness, I did my best to provide a sense of hope, and they did the very same for me. I do not know what compelled me to do this, but I felt like it was my responsibility to reach out to the other patients when the circumstances were appropriate. I do not know if this type of leadership stemmed from being the captain of my high school swim team, but I truly wanted to make a connection with them and their families because I felt, from my own experience, that there was always that chance I could help motivate them. I talked to them, said prayers for them, and tried to give them hope. While doing so, I realized that I was also giving myself hope for my own future.

When I was released to go back home, I immediately started to participate in outpatient therapy several times a week. After spending a few months in a wheelchair, I took baby steps to walk on my own with a walker, then a cane, and then with some help from my parents on each side of me. It was a miracle that I could walk again, but I wanted to push even further to not only walk, but run. After I accomplished that, I wanted to get back in the pool again. The human spirit is an amazing thing. After a few lung tests, I was able to go in the pool a little bit each week.

Before the accident I had three short-term goals after graduating from high school: go to college, swim on the team, and one day compete in an Ironman triathlon, which is the most difficult and challenging single-day athletic event in the world. The Ironman is a long-distance event that consists of a 2.4-mile swim in the ocean, followed by a 112-mile bike ride, and then a 26.2-mile marathon run. To say that this is a long race is an understatement, not to mention that you are given only seventeen hours to complete this 140.6-mile event. I grew up watching this race on TV, and as intense as it looked, it was on my radar to complete one day.

After a few months of transitioning from dog-paddling to swimming in the pool, I decided I was going to pursue my dreams despite my injuries. I began my freshman year in college a year after leaving the ICU, and I accomplished my second goal by swimming on the team.

Two years later, I was given the opportunity to participate in my third goal, the Ironman. Up until that point in my recovery, I was in college, on the swim team, and living the life of a typical college student. My life was returning to normal, but the healing was not complete. I still felt like there was something missing, and deep in my heart I knew that it would take something as extreme as the Ironman to complete the recovery.

On October 13, 2007, I had the chance to complete the healing at the Ironman World Championship in Kona, Hawaii. It was an incredibly emotional day for my parents and me because we had gone through so much over the past few years. After almost fifteen hours of swimming, biking, and running, I walked slowly up to the finish line, turned around to take in the surreal moment, and then I put my arms up in victory. I gave my parents the biggest hug that I had ever given them. I made it, I had reached the finish line. In that moment, on that Ironman finish line in the late evening of October 13, I was fully healed. My recovery was complete.

Suggestions for Health Care Providers and/or Patient's Family:

- Before you interact with patients in a situation similar to Brian's, reflect on how you could help ease the pain of a suffering family as they work through the initial shock.
- Always treat the patient as a person and not just as an injured body.
- The family wants answers on the patient's condition, and although you sometimes cannot give any answers, you can take the time to address their concerns.

Reflective Questions for Health Care Providers (write your answers in Part Five):

1) How often do you reflect on the patient's experience? The family's experience?
2) Imagine being in Brian's shoes when he started to regain consciousness. How would you feel?
3) Imagine the feeling that Brian's parents had when they received the phone call that Brian was in critical condition, and the feeling they had when they saw him in the recovery room for the first time. What thoughts would be going through your mind at this point in time?

4) Imagine being one of Brian's care providers when he first arrived at the hospital. What is one particular thing that you could do to help his loved ones adjust to the shock of the situation?

5) As a care provider, how do you personally find hope in a seemingly hopeless situation (i.e., stepping back from the "Oh wow, they are really sick" moment to take the appropriate steps to treat the patient)?

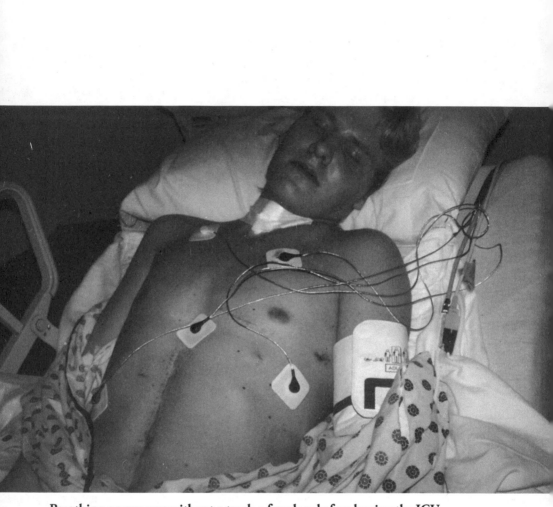

Breathing on my own without a trach a few days before leaving the ICU.

CHAPTER 2

A VOICE FOR THE VOICELESS

When I returned home from the Hawaii Ironman, I reflected on the promise that I made to myself while sitting in the wheelchair at my rehab center. Now that I was healed, it was time for me to show gratitude for the new life I had been given. I was on a mission to give back.

I started this journey by reaching out to my local Red Cross affiliate—the Red Cross Greater Chesapeake & Potomac Blood Services region, based in Baltimore. I shared my story with them and asked what I could do to help raise awareness on the importance of blood donation. They contacted me a few weeks later and I presented my story at a board of directors meeting, attended a few blood drives, and did a couple interviews with local television stations and newspapers. With all that I had been through over the years, I was finally starting to see that I could help others by sharing my experiences and becoming a voice for the voiceless.

After a few months of volunteering, my story traveled throughout the Maryland area and received attention from the National Headquarters of the American Red Cross in Washington, DC. From there, the story quickly spread throughout the Mid-Atlantic, along the East Coast, and then across the country. What started out as just saying thank you at a couple of local meetings transformed into speaking on behalf of blood recipients on a national level. I was no longer just attending blood drives, but I was hosting my own—Iron Heart Red Cross blood drives—all over the country. I was no longer just doing interviews in newspapers, but I was writing articles in national publications such as *The Washington Post* and *The Huffington Post*. I was speaking on behalf of blood donation in regional and national television interviews, at universities, and in various auditoriums and conference halls each week.

Since 2007, I have volunteered a great deal of my time with the American Red Cross, and my proudest accomplishment as a volunteer was to go back and donate blood at the hospital that saved my life. While I sat in my chair waiting to donate, I thought about where my blood was going. Whom would it help? A mother? A father? A son or daughter? A baby? An adult? A person battling cancer, a sickle-cell anemia patient, or maybe a person involved in a car accident? A chill ran down my spine as I thought about the lifesaving power that blood donation has for the people who receive it, and I knew in that moment, whomever it would be given to, it would help improve that person's life.

I give credit where it is due, and it has been an honor to volunteer for an organization that played such a vital role in my recovery. When I needed it, the American Red Cross was there, with thirty-six blood transfusions and thirteen plasma treatments that helped save my life. There are forty-nine people who took one hour of their time to help save the life of someone they would never have a chance to know. I would not be alive today if it were not for these selfless people, whom I do not know and will never meet. Volunteer blood donors made this possible. By giving just a little bit of their time, blood donors gave me the chance at a lifetime.

With this life that I have been given, I have been an advocate not only for blood donation, but also for health care and patient safety. In the same way that I wanted to acknowledge my appreciation to the Red Cross and their blood donors, I also wanted to reach out and show my gratitude to people who chose to work in the field of health care.

The first place that I wanted to visit and say thank you to was my hospital. After this event, I was then invited to represent my hospital by speaking at an annual meeting for the Maryland Hospital Association. My story and message of gratitude to care providers rapidly spread across the nation, similar to the way that it did with the Red Cross.

As a health care advocate, I have traveled the country and spoken at annual meetings for many state hospital associations, at dozens of health care leadership conferences, and at several annual conventions and medical symposiums. I have proudly given over one hundred keynote presentations at various health care events whose attendees included hospital leaders, doctors, nurses, EMS providers, patient-safety experts, patient-experience experts, military medical personnel, nursing home personnel, medical suppliers, physical therapists, and nursing school students. I have represented the patient experience in meetings and discussions with governors, senators, mayors, and members of the US House of Representatives.

From the East Coast to the West Coast, from my hospital all the way to the White House in our nation's capital, I have served as a living example of the extraordinary work that care providers do every day. During my travels, I have collaborated with several world-renowned health-care institutions on projects related to patient and family engagement in the hospital setting. After I was invited by Dr. Peter Pronovost to give the keynote presentation at the 2012 Johns Hopkins Patient Safety Summit, he requested that I also serve as a volunteer patient advocate to work with him and his team at the Armstrong Institute for Patient Safety and Quality at Johns Hopkins. It meant a lot to me that I was able to work with them on "Project Emerge," which consisted of a technologically innovative electronic tablet that improves communication among the patient, family, and care team in the hospital setting. I am currently studying at Johns Hopkins University for a Master of Arts in Communication with a concentration in Health Communication, along with a Master of Business Administration with a concentration in Health Care Management.

While speaking as a health care advocate, I met a lot of amazing people who had overcome a lot in their lives. It was these interactions that inspired me to publish my first book, *Iron Heart*, in 2009. I began writing journals for therapeutic reasons when I was released from the hospital, and I was motivated to publish those personal reflections with the hope they would land in the hands of a person going through an adverse situation similar to mine. My journey has truly come full circle over the years, and my mission to make an impact with my background is only just beginning.

It is always an emotional experience for me to reflect on my time in the hospital. I give a piece of my heart and soul in every chapter of this book. The content on every page represents my appreciation for the amazing people like you—for the work that you do—who save people like me.

Suggestions for Health Care Providers and/or Patient's Family:

- Help keep your patients focused on the positive things that they have going for them (they are alive, people believe in them, you are supporting them, etc.).

- Help keep the family members focused on the positive aspects of the patient's recovery process.

- Approach any conversation with a family member in a manner that helps put that person at ease, as difficult as this may be sometimes. Even the tone of a voice can be significant.

- Showing sincerity and empathy goes a long way with the patient and his or her family.

Reflective Questions for Health Care Providers (write your answers in Part Five):

1) How would you feel if you were no longer able to physically complete the activities of daily living?

2) How do you physically and mentally prepare a patient and family to transition from acute care to rehabilitation?

3) When a patient is very focused on the negative aspects of his or her situation, how can you help that patient focus on finding the strength to keep striving toward making improvements?

4) After you discharge a patient, do you wonder how he or she is doing as that patient navigates through the health care system and recovery process?

5) How often do you hear how your patients are doing after they have been discharged? How does it make you feel knowing that you contributed to their recovery?

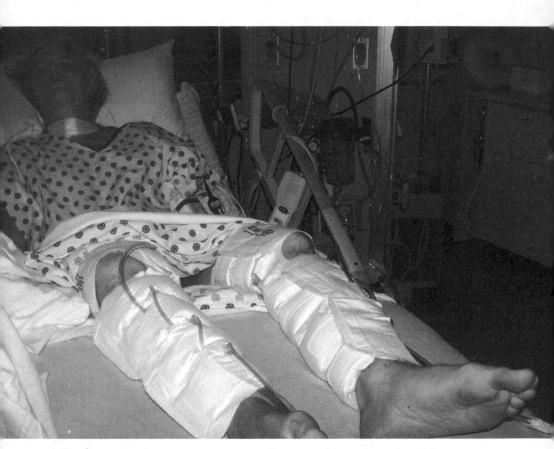

When it came to the recovery process, progress was slow and consisted of continuous setbacks.

CHAPTER 3

BRIAN'S WEBSITE

Details in the first two chapters briefly summarized the recovery process, which can be read in full detail in my first book, *Iron Heart*.

In this chapter, we will take a closer look at the recovery process by reading firsthand accounts from a website that provided updates on my condition. These entries give brief insight into the daily struggles and improvements that patients and their families experience in the hospital room. I present all of my parents' entries unabridged to illustrate the intense rising and falling action of life in the ICU; you can skim a selection of entries, but I recommend you read every one to get a full picture of the patient (and family) experience.

As soon as the news spread that I was in the hospital in critical condition, my parents started to receive an endless number of phone calls. People started to come to our house and visit the hospital to hear updates on my condition and offer to help my parents in any way that they could. The outpouring of support meant a lot to my parents, but it became overwhelming for them. They had to relive the nightmarish details every time they gave an update on my status, which was very grim during the first few days. Mom and Dad were still in shock with everything that was going on, and they were not really sure what to do in this situation. My health was slipping so fast that they made the decision to start letting relatives and close friends say their final good-byes.

As I made it through the first few days, my family thought it would be helpful to create a website to keep everyone updated on my daily health status, from the day of the accident all the way through rehab. Not only was this an effective and far-reaching method to keep everyone updated on how I was doing, but it was helpful for my parents because they no longer had to recount the details several times a day.

Brian's Page was quickly established, and my parents were encouraged to write a daily summary on the long drive home from the hospital. My uncle would enter the short paragraphs on the "Daily Update" section of the site to keep everyone updated and to help them process and cope with the anguish they were facing each day.

In reality, the overviews published on the website were very mild compared to the truth of what was actually happening. The journal entries were geared toward my peers, teenagers. They noted positive things that were happening each day, rather than all the depressing and gruesome aspects of the procedures, tests, and constant setbacks. Writing the overviews gave family and friends hope, and also helped to keep my parents focused on a positive outcome.

Daily Update

7/6: Brian arrives at Prince George's Hospital Center. He has multiple fractures to the left side of his body and his pelvis is broken. He has lost 60 percent of his blood. The main concern when he was brought into shock trauma is that his heart was pushed to the opposite side of his chest by the impact of the crash. He was taken immediately into surgery and the damage to the heart was successfully repaired. Unfortunately, his spleen has to be removed. There is much concern as to the possibility of brain damage, but the doctors must wait to perform a CAT scan until his blood pressure is stabilized. There is a question as to whether or not there is additional internal bleeding. He is heavily sedated, and becomes very agitated when he begins to regain consciousness. He is on a ventilator. Hospital personnel are cautiously hopeful.

7/7: This was a long day. The doctors were able to perform both the CAT scan and angiogram. Much to the relief of the family, the CAT scan showed no evidence of trauma to the brain. The angiogram showed no additional bleeding from the heart. He is still on life support. We do know that he has significant trauma to many other organs in addition to the heart. His lungs are badly bruised and his left kidney has been fractured, similar to a bone being broken, but the kidney is working properly. Also, his body is becoming extremely swollen due to the treatments he is receiving. Because of Brian's strong build and blond hair, his critical care team nicknamed him "Thor" after the Norse god of thunder. They think this is also appropriate based on how hard his body is fighting to get well. When they caught a glimpse of his lightning bolt tattoo, they knew they picked the right name.

7/7: Late evening. Doctors were concerned that there was additional blood collecting in the abdomen and decided to operate again. They found and successfully repaired a tear in his diaphragm. At this stage of treatment, the doctors like to see how he will respond to less sedation. He becomes agitated when he begins to regain consciousness, but this is a good sign at this point.

7/8: The reports today have slightly improved. Brian had a good night and the swelling has gone down. He is looking more like himself. A renal specialist is scheduled to take a look at the kidney today. Joanne (Mom) and Garth (Dad) were able to see Brian again this afternoon and they were thrilled to see not only how well he looked, but also how pleased the doctors and nurses were with his progress. The renal specialist shared positive news that Brian's damaged kidney should recover on its own. There is still concern regarding the lungs, which were very badly bruised. While Brian is able to breathe on his own, they have decided to keep him on the ventilator so his body does not have to work so hard. The doctors are pleased with the progress, and for the first time, immediate family was granted visiting privileges this evening. Please note: at this time only immediate family can see him.

7/9: Reports from the hospital today were better even though Brian remains in critical condition. He had a good night. His blood count decreased as a result of the kidney dialysis machine he is hooked up to so he required one unit of blood. The day continued with fewer problems. More family members were able to see him this morning. His parents were happy to see more improvement and the swelling continues to go down. The kidneys are functioning, so the kidney dialysis machine was removed, and a drainage tube was removed from his heart. He continues to be stable throughout the day. Since day one he has no cuts on his head or face and the shaggy hair is flowing (you know Brian and his hair!). The doctors also ordered a bigger bed. His feet would dangle over the bottom of the bed if his legs were straighter.

To all Brian's friends: First we would like to thank all of you for your thoughts and prayers. A lot of you may be wondering how Brian's morning was prior to the accident. He got up that morning at 8:30; he had stayed up late the night before making his 311 mix CD in preparation for the concert. Had a bowl of cereal and a nutrition bar (you all know Mr. Healthy). He did his ab work-out regime (Dad found the tape in the VCR), then went to the track to run and came home to change for the pool to train for the St. Mary's College Swim Team. He called up his dad to let him know he was on the way to the pool, which he normally does not do. Dad said, "Have a good practice—proud of you." Brian then called his mom to let her know he was on the way to the pool, and to remind her to stop by St. Mary's College to change a class on his schedule, which is easy to do because she works at the naval base near the school.

7/10: Another stable night. Brian's coach, teacher, and mentor stopped by to visit him. Mom and Dad were very happy because they know how much he means to Brian.

Late afternoon: Concern about some additional problems with Brian's lungs. More testing is planned. Due to this new development, Brian's doctors have decided to deny visitors at this time. Please respect the decision and continue to check here for updates.

7/11: A very rough day. The lungs are a concern. Pneumonia and blood clots were mentioned, so a chest X-ray was taken and a CAT scan was performed. Both tests came back negative. Brian was trying to wake up and was very agitated. The doctors are trying to find the correct combination of pain medications. He is still chemically unconscious and on life support. One of Brian's trauma doctors is a former football player. Every time he sees Brian he tells Mom and Dad that he cannot believe Brian did not play football. The doctor went up to the head of Brian's bed and yelled to him, "Hey, Brian, how ya doing, man? Give me a thumbs-up. You can do it!" Brian struggled, but he got the message and gave the signal. When Mom saw that thumb come up, she was able to cry some happy tears for a change.

To all Brian's friends: The visit with Brian's coach yesterday proved a milestone for Brian's parents. Even though he is unconscious, when his coach asked Brian if he wanted him to go, he shook his head "no." He then asked Brian, "Do you want me to stay?" Brian squeezed his hand and nodded "yes," with tears welling up in his closed eyes.

7/12: A long day. Brian's fever was high. His parents brought in a fan for his room to help with his fever. The doctors are still trying to come up with the right combination of pain medications. Brian became a little rambunctious in between doses and pulled out one of his chest tubes, but by midday he seemed to calm down. He looked comfortable. The shades were closed, the lights were off, and the fan produced a cool breeze—a little bit of relief for his mom and dad.

Early evening: Doctors found a blood clot in the groin area where the kidney dialysis machine was attached several days earlier. Brian had to return to the operating room so the doctors could insert a type of filter, an umbrella-shaped device that catches the blood clots and prevents them from traveling to the lungs. The procedure went well and Brian was back in his room and asleep after a few hours.

To all Brian's friends: His parents are continually hearing his nurses, doctors, police, and others involved praising the fact that Brian came in without any trace of alcohol, drugs, or tobacco in his system. They commented how this is almost unheard of in this type of situation. Along with his youth, his healthy diet, regular workout regimen, and active participation in sports are all working in his favor.

7/13: A quiet day. The pain medication was kicking in. Brian was a lot calmer today even though his fever was very high. The nurses had him under a cooling blanket with ice packs strategically placed in various areas. His neck collar was removed today and he was sleeping with his head to the side, facing the fan. In the early evening he went for a CAT scan for the chest, abdomen, and pelvis. The results will be back in the morning.

To all Brian's friends: The swim coach at St. Mary's College called today. All of Brian's college-related materials were due by the end of this month. Much to the relief of his parents, the coach has kindly offered to take care of all these details. Brian's parents also received a phone call from the director of the indoor pool that Brian was swimming at on the day of the accident. The director called to let them know that he was the last person to see Brian before the accident. Brian had stepped into his office, very happy and excited, to tell him that his training was going well and he was looking forward to attending St. Mary's in August.

7/14: Another quiet day. Brian was still fighting the infection, which caused his fever to go up and down. Knowing the many problems Brian was going to face, the doctors told his parents in the beginning that this would be a roller-coaster ride. The director of the ICU said his CAT scan came back OK, except for a dilated bladder, which they will keep an eye on. They also mentioned the possibility of performing a tracheotomy and removing the current breathing tube. This not only would be more comfortable for Brian, but also would pose less risk of infection. The doctors said that we are "not out of the woods yet."

7/15: Today was better, worse, and then better. Mom and Dad were happy to see how Brian looked this morning. He had color in his face and the swelling had gone down even more. Doctors took out the second of the two chest tubes today (remember that Brian removed the other one himself several days ago). What we did not know when that happened was that it was actually stitched in. The nurses say that he can be quite the little beast. When he woke between doses and got feisty, which indicates that he is in pain, his parents heard *the nurses call for one of the young and athletic employees to help get Brian settled. Later, he received two more units of blood, which they say is normal for the type of trauma he has sustained. His trauma surgeon says he will wait one more day before making the decision to perform the tracheotomy, but he is expecting Brian will need to have the surgery by Saturday. Nurses said Brian can finally have some music, and you all know Brian and his music. They think this will help him as he begins to regain consciousness.*

7/16: Rough night, quiet day. Brian was more deeply sedated today because the nurses had a difficult time with him last night. They said he literally tried to climb out of the bed and pull out more of his tubes. The nurses maintain that this is normal for anyone in his condition. Waking up between doses and finding yourself tied down, with machines all around and attached to your body, is very frightening. They are continually surprised at how strong he is when he begins to wake. He even has mittens on his hands to inhibit his ability to grasp onto anything and potentially pull it out. He did receive two more units of blood, which is normal for trauma patients. He will be going back for surgery, possibly tomorrow, for the tracheotomy. The doctors say that while this is still considered life support, it is more comfortable than the breathing tube he currently must endure. The nurses turned on the TV today to keep him company. He is missing all the Olympic trials in his favorite sports, but these events are being taped and the sports sections are being saved for him. Please continue to respect the doctors' no-visitation policy.

7/17: Quiet day. Brian was on heavy sedation today. The tracheotomy is scheduled for 8 a.m. Otherwise, no real news.

7/18: Long day. Brian had the tracheotomy this morning at 8 a.m. and the surgery went well. They have moved the feeding tube to Brian's nose. The tracheotomy replaces the ventilator tube that went down his throat, so there is no longer anything in his mouth. He is still very heavily sedated because they are trying to keep him calm. He still has fever, infection, and some swelling. He is not in the "safe zone" yet.

7/19: Scary day. Brian was so swollen he looked like a sumo wrestler. The doctors surmised this was his body's reaction to yesterday's surgery. He had another CAT scan early this evening and thankfully the results came back showing no problems. He is still heavily sedated to keep him calm. Hopefully tomorrow will be a better day.

7/20: Long day. Brian was still heavily sedated. Mom and Dad brought in his CD player today and started things off with a little reggae. Since he just came back from Jamaica, maybe some familiar sounds might be soothing. He has gone from sumo-wrestler to professional-wrestler size. Pneumonia has set in, which the doctors say is another stage in the process.

7/21: Really rough day. Brian was still fighting infection and pneumonia. Around midday the fluid from his lungs clogged the trach tube. The doctors and nurses had to work fast to get another breathing tube down through his mouth and into his chest. A specialist then had to come in to vacuum the fluid out of his lungs. Brian will be back in surgery tomorrow to have a larger tracheotomy tube inserted.

7/22: Long day. Today Brian had the surgery to insert the larger tracheostomy tube. The surgery went fine, but he is back on 100 percent life support. His fever remains very high, as he is still fighting infection. He has been chemically paralyzed to keep him calm and still. The doctors believe this will not only aid him with his breathing, but also help his lungs heal. The roller coaster of ups and downs is still moving. Brian's trauma surgeon used another example of the healing process today when he said it is like a plane that takes off and attempts to get to the right altitude, but hits some bumps on the way to reaching the calm air at the higher elevation. Brian is still flying through the turbulence.

To all Brian's friends: Brian was switched to a new bed today. This bed completely tilts from side to side; at times it can turn Brian sideways, facing the wall, even though his back is flat on the bed. The purpose is to keep the fluid in his lungs moving and help him fight the pneumonia. Maybe he will dream that he is riding the big waves. You all know Brian and how he loves going to the beach.

7/23: Another long day. Brian remained very heavily sedated, and is still fighting pneumonia. His fever is still up and down. He received more blood today and continues to be chemically paralyzed. He is flowing from side to side on his bed, and today the nurses increased the tilt angle. It looks like something from a science fiction movie.

7/24: Long day, once again. Brian continued to be heavily sedated. He had to receive two more units of blood today. His temperature actually dropped to 99 degrees, which was the high point of the day.

7/25: This was a frightening day. Brian is being weaned off the paralysis medication and has started to wake, off and on. The first visit went OK, but the second was a bit rough. The scary part is watching him try to cough with the trach. The nurses quickly suction, but the fear of the tube getting clogged again is still there, and he is once again agitated. His mom fell apart today, but his dad remained strong. Dad said to Brian, "Dad's here. If you know Daddy's here, squeeze my hand. Calm down or the nurses will make me leave." Brian then calmed down and squeezed Dad's hand. The highlight of the day was when one of the nurses washed and combed his hair and gave him a shave. She said, "That baby face of his needed to be cleaned up." Brian's aunt has been talking to the helicopter crew and fire department personnel to thank them for their efforts. The helicopter crew said they want Brian to come see them when he is well and they will take him for a ride over DC. On a good note, his parents finally solved a mystery that started the day of the accident. On that evening, a police officer called in to the trauma unit and spoke to the director of nursing. He said he could not sleep until he found out how Brian was. He also wanted to tell all the personnel who were caring for Brian that he was a "good boy." The nurses continued to talk to Brian's parents about this policeman, but could not remember his name. He turned out to be a police officer from McDonough High School. His parents are truly touched by what he said and did. Thanks also to Brian's school principal for all his help and thoughtfulness.

7/26: Stressful day. Brian's condition remains the same; no real change. Doctors are trying to find the source of infection. They are looking at the gall-bladder and the liver. He was sent to Nuclear Radiology at 2 p.m. to check these organs, but the tests came back inconclusive. They repeated the same tests this evening, and they will do an MRI in the morning before considering surgery.

7/27: Three weeks today. Brian is still heavily sedated, swollen, and now once again on the medicine to keep him paralyzed. His nurse said that his metabolism is so strong that it takes a large dose to keep him down. They also had to put a chest tube in again to drain fluid from his body. His trauma surgeon has decided to take him back into surgery tomorrow at 8:50 a.m. to try to determine the site of infection. He believes it is probably the gallbladder, in which case the organ will be removed.

7/28: Change of plans. His trauma surgeon decided to wait another day before performing the surgery and chose to order a CAT scan instead. He does not want to operate again unless absolutely necessary. The results came back, but did not show anything significant. Brian is still heavily sedated.

To all Brian's friends: Brian has a new roommate today, but this time it is another young person, a seventeen-year-old girl who has also been involved in a serious car accident. No lecture, but Brian's parents would just like to say, please be careful driving. It is not just drugs and alcohol that cause accidents—they can happen to anyone, both girls and boys, young and old. You have so much to live for and enjoy. Please be safe.

7/29: Quiet day. The ICU director took Brian off the paralysis medicine, but he is still heavily sedated. His care team has decided again to hold off on the surgery.

To all Brian's friends: For those of you attending the 311 concert, please enjoy it for Brian. He was really looking forward to the show, as 311 is one of his favorite bands.

7/30: Quiet day. Brian's parents are holding their breath; another day has gone by without surgery. He is still heavily sedated, on life support, and his temperature is up.

7/31: Quiet day. All information from yesterday remains essentially the same today. Brian sometimes begins to move around slightly, then goes back to sleep. The sedation keeps him from getting agitated.

8/1: Quiet day. Brian's condition today was very much like yesterday. His trauma surgeon came by to check in and requested another CAT scan to be given after midnight tonight. Not sure what we are in for tomorrow. Brian's parents received a nice letter from the superintendent of Charles County Schools. Brian enjoyed his time at McDonough High School; he worked hard in academics and he played hard in athletics. His parents were truly touched that someone at this level would take the time to send a letter. It was very much appreciated.

8/2: Quiet day. Brian remained heavily sedated. The trauma surgeon continues to hold off on the surgery. He is OK with the results of the CAT scan for the time being. As we have come to learn, in trauma, it is all minute by minute, hour by hour, day by day. The trauma surgeon has commented that he does not like to cut unless absolutely necessary. He also determined that Brian has a sinus infection and that most swimmers carry this condition. He has requested an ENT (Ear, Nose, and Throat) specialist to check on him. The feeding tube has been moved from Brian's nose to his throat and, even though unconscious, you can tell he finds this uncomfortable. We will see what tomorrow will bring.

8/3: One month today. No real news, but no news is good news.

To all Brian's friends: Mom and Dad received a nice surprise today when they returned home from the hospital. They opened a large mailing envelope to find a guitar pick, sticker, and autographed picture from the band 311. The band signed the picture: "Brian—We're wishing you strength and positivity. All the best, 311." We don't know who contacted the band's management company, but thank you to that person.

8/4: Lots of action today. More tomorrow. Brian's fever went back up to nearly 102 degrees last night. The trauma surgeon has decided that the surgery he has been putting off is now necessary. He will perform the procedure tomorrow to check for the source of the infection, clean him out, and possibly remove the gallbladder. Another development has been a buildup of fluid around Brian's heart. A cardiac surgeon will double-team with Brian's trauma surgeon during the procedure, and they will install a drainage tube to reduce this excess fluid.

8/5: Long day. Brian had his surgery today. The trauma surgeon said he washed the inside of Brian's chest because he had a buildup of fluid. He also decided to remove the gallbladder. The cardiac surgeon drained the fluid from around the heart and inserted a drainage tube. Both surgeons reported that the surgery went well.

8/6: Quiet day. Brian is still heavily medicated since his surgery. More of the swelling has gone down due to the draining of the fluid around the heart. His temperature was still up and down.

8/7: Quiet day; same as yesterday. The nurses turned down his sedation this morning to check Brian's response. Even though he is chemically unconscious, he did get agitated. His respiratory therapist asked him to open his eyes for her, and he did for a second, then closed them. They said that was a good response. If only Brian's fever would break.

8/8: Big day. The nurses turned down his sedation for the two o'clock visit so Mom and Dad could see him open his eyes, and he did! He opened his baby blues, but you can tell he is heavily medicated. As Dad spoke quietly, Brian looked at him for about ten minutes. Dad is still doing better than Mom. Brian then fell back to sleep. His temperature is still up and down.

8/9: Hard day. The ICU director is waking Brian slowly. His eyes opened and closed more often today. Several times he woke and looked terrified, even though he was still heavily medicated. He would look at and listen to Dad, and Dad was able to calm him down. A nurse agreed with the doctors that this is all good, but to Brian and his parents it is sheer terror. The temperature is still up and down. The white blood count is getting closer to the normal range: Friday it was 21; today it was down to 12. Normal is around 10.

8/10: Five weeks today. The care team continues to wean Brian off the drugs, and he is beginning to get feisty. His arms are tied down and his legs are probably next. This is going to be another rough phase, especially for his parents. However, everyone is saying it is a good phase. Mom is already running out of the room after ten minutes, fearing she will fall apart, and leaving Dad to calm Brian down. One of the hospital employees keeps trying to cheer Mom up by joking that she is "going to get her crying belt out" if she sees her running out of the room one more time. Mom was very touched this afternoon when she did feel the need to leave the room and this employee came looking for her; it was a great comfort. Brian also got another bed today. It is huge. A combination of an air and water bed. His nurse got him situated, and then somehow Brian got the feeding tube out of his throat. She tried to put it back down, but he threw up all over the new bed, the sheets, and the nurse. She left, changed her clothes, and came back to continue working on him. We are blessed to have such an excellent medical team watching over Brian. In fact, the entire hospital staff—from the parking lot attendants to the front desk personnel at the lobby and the trauma unit, from the security guards to the cafeteria workers, from the maintenance people to all the doctors and nurses, even the people working in the business office—have shown such kindness to Brian and his parents that it is truly overwhelming. Even the ICU director, a very serious professional, calls Brian his buddy now.

8/11: Rough day. The nurse said Brian's vital signs are becoming stable, and she is letting him wake up more today. However, the process of weaning him off the drugs is not easy. He is going through withdrawal now, which is very difficult to watch. If poor Brian only knew, because he has always been so anti-drug. His respiratory therapist was back today, and Brian seems to listen to her. Mom and Dad call her Brian's guardian angel. Brian had to be moved to another area of the hospital to have his feeding tube replaced. Transporting him requires a whole team of people, and his respiratory therapist went with the team on his road trip. During the procedure, Brian became agitated and the respiratory therapist and several nurses were able to calm him down. Mom and Dad say the nurses who take care of Brian are excellent. They call him their baby, little brother, or grandson depending on which nurse it is. They sincerely care for him. Dad was able to calm him again, but the look of terror in Brian's eyes is heartbreaking. Dad is still doing a great job, but he lost Mom a few times today when she disappeared. Sometimes watching is just too much to bear.

8/12: Smile day. A nurse called this morning to say Brian had an interesting night. He was a bit feisty, and did have some more vomiting, which is a symptom of withdrawal. However, she said he calmed down afterward. It does hurt him with the stitches, feeding tube, and trach tube. As Mom and Dad were leaving for the hospital, the respiratory therapist called to say that he was following commands. She asked him if he wanted to hear some music and he shook his head "yes." When his parents arrived at the hospital, the nurses said he had given them a smile. Then, Mom and Dad went in and he gave them a smile. In came the rest of his care team, and Brian smiled at each one of them. He even tried to lift his hands to shake theirs, but of course they are still tied down. He is a true gentleman. Someone even said, "He is an amazing kid. With the hell he is going through, he still has his manners." Brian is still on life support, so he cannot talk. This frustrates and scares him.

He still has that look of terror and gets a bit weepy when his eyes open. It is still a scary time, as we all know by now. However, Brian did seem to have a moment of peace: as Dad turned on the radio, a Fleetwood Mac song began playing. They saw his face immediately relax, with his eyes showing a sense of contentment. One of the drugs that Brian is being weaned off is ten times stronger than morphine, which is why the withdrawal phase is so difficult. The drugs that saved his life are now the demons he is trying to fight.

8/13: Calm day. Brian is still going through withdrawal, but he is a bit calmer today. They are using methadone to take the edge off the withdrawal. They are also giving him another medication to help with the nausea. When the ICU director walked in this morning, Brian's face lit up. He is still following commands and smiling. He had a heart test this afternoon to check if there was any additional fluid buildup since the surgery. The test results will be back tomorrow. The nurses also gave Brian a spa day. They washed his hair, put Vaseline on his lips, washed his face, and got him all cleaned up. They had an ocean scene and beach sounds on TV today to keep him calm. They also requested that Mom and Dad spend extra time with Brian today because their presence helps to keep him calm. As they were leaving after their first visit this morning, Brian opened his eyes. He put his left hand up for Mom to hold, then he put his right hand up for Dad to hold. He seemed to be saying, "You guys are not going anywhere!" After having a hard time for the past couple of days, Mom was able to stay in Brian's room for the entire hour during all three visits. A nurse called tonight to tell Mom and Dad that she had asked Brian if he wanted to watch the Olympics. Looking excited, he shook his head "yes." He put his head up to watch TV. He is not alert enough to remember what he sees, but he can enjoy it for the moment.

8/14: *Rough day. No real news. However, the withdrawal has been causing extreme shaking. Nurses say this is normal and that it is all a part of the withdrawal process.*

8/15: *Sleepy day. Brian is still going through the withdrawal phase with all the shaking and sweating, and was not as coherent today. This might take a while because he is being weaned off the heavy drugs very slowly. He slept most of the day and we should get the results of the heart test tomorrow. Mom and Dad have finally been given the go-ahead to check out some rehabilitation facilities.*

8/16: *Terribly rough day. A nurse called last night and she said that she is getting him in a chair today because she wants to get things rolling. When Mom and Dad arrived, Brian was in a hospital chair, but he is still in the withdrawal stage with lots of shaking, sweating, and coughing. The ICU director is trying to further wean Brian off the drugs. They want him to be more coherent, and he was not at all coherent today. All the nurses love Brian. He has become well known all over the hospital. Various hospital personnel keep coming by to check on him. They say he is going through the withdrawal phase and he is doing OK, but to Mom and Dad it is still very frightening.*

8/17: *Six weeks today. Brian had a difficult night followed by another rough day. His fever shot up to 104 degrees and his white blood count went up to 33. A normal count is 10 and Brian's had been hovering around 11. The high white count indicates infection. Brian was back under the cooling blanket (40 degrees) that had been removed from his room days ago. The ICU director ordered CAT scans of Brian's brain, chest, abdomen, and pelvis. Mom and Dad arrived at the hospital early to give consent for the tests and to see Brian. He rolled by on his hallway road trip with four nurses. He does like the ladies, but he has no idea how many he has looking out for him. We received the CAT scan results in the early afternoon, and they all looked OK. The medical team thinks the rise in temperature and white blood count is due to the withdrawal, but infection is another possibility. His sinuses are still acting up, and Brian may have a few more rocky days because he is being weaned off even more of the drugs. By the time Mom and Dad left tonight, he was sweating profusely. Everyone is hoping that this is a sign that the fever is breaking. He is still not very coherent, but he showed some signs of emotion today. When dad changed the CD in the stereo, he asked Brian, "If this is OK, close your eyes." Up to this point, Brian had been staring blankly into space. When Dad asked this question, Brian closed his eyes. Mom and Dad are thrilled with even the tiniest response. The nurse even let them stay a little bit over the time limit because she said it seems to comfort him. Everyone says, "The kid's got to get a break."*

8/18: Long day. Brian remains in the withdrawal phase, staring into space, and is still not very coherent. The ICU director is really trying to turn things around and get him off the drugs. There were only a few responses from Brian today. The nurse said she wanted to shift him around a bit, and Brian seemed to try to help her as she moved him into different positions. The last visit was a comfort to Mom and Dad. As they were sitting with Brian, the ICU director, director of nursing, and trauma surgeon explained that they were going to try a different antibiotic to combat the possible infection. A good note is that the white blood count was down today, from 33 to 17. The temperature was still up, but not as high, and they have turned off the cooling blanket.

8/19: Better day. The nurse called this morning to say Brian had a good night. The ICU director was back to see Brian again last night and asked Brian if he would like to watch the Olympics. Brian gave his first response in five days when he nodded "yes." When Mom and Dad arrived in the morning, the curtains were drawn in Brian's room because the physical therapist was working with him. The nurses said that he was giving faint responses. The respiratory therapist even tested his breathing for four hours. The Ear, Nose, and Throat (ENT) specialist came in and was pleased to tell Mom and Dad that the sinuses were almost clear and surgery would not be necessary. Brian looked at the ENT with a faint smile, and tried to lift his arm so they could shake hands. He could not quite get his hand in the correct position, but the ENT helped him. Next came the doctor in charge of the physical therapy department. She greeted Brian and asked him to do a few things that included sticking out his tongue, wiggling his toes, and lifting his right arm. He was able to complete all his tasks. His temperature is now down in the 99 to 100 degree range and there was also good news about the white blood count. Remember that a high white count indicates infection and a normal count is less than 10. Today the white count was 9.6. The swelling is all gone. He is still sweating profusely, but not shaking as bad. He seems to be awake more, but still in a fog. The last five days were very bad. The director of nursing was right when she said that we would be riding a roller coaster. It was thundering this evening, another reminder of Thor (Brian's nickname from the nurses). Early into Brian's ordeal, his coach brought him a Thor comic book, which hangs in his hospital room. Mom took it off the wall and showed it to Brian, not knowing it was about to thunder. It is also Thursday, which originally comes from "Thor's Day."

8/20: No real news tonight; same as yesterday. Brian's responses seem to be a little quicker. They are starting to test his breathing capacity.

To all Brian's friends: The dietitian started Brian on protein feedings to help increase his weight. You all know Mr. Healthy and his protein drinks!

8/21: *Slow day. Brian is gradually waking up and he continues to respond a little more. The responses are very faint, although he tried to give a few smiles to the female nurses when they came in. His eyes seem to be open more and he stayed awake longer. His breathing continues to be tested and his body is very weak. His muscle mass is not what it was, but the nurses explained that he will eventually get it back. Dad asked if he wanted him to bring in his hand exerciser and he nodded "yes." But Dad said the barbells may have to wait! The ICU director came in today and tried to motivate Brian to wake up. He told Mom and Dad to keep him awake during visiting hours. Even though he is a doctor, he came in like a coach. They asked Brian if he would like to have any friends or family come to visit him. He responded with an almost frightened look, shaking his head "no." They then asked, "How about when you are feeling better?" He nodded "yes."*

To all Brian's friends: The nurse asked Mom and Dad about trimming Brian's hair. After washing it, she had tried to style it like it was in the picture, but she could not get it to look quite right. Mom and Dad asked Brian if he wanted a haircut. His baby blues opened quickly and he shook his head "no!" Even his eyebrows moved on that one. The saga of Brian's hair continues!

8/22: *Really bad day. Brian has started to exhibit some different symptoms apparently related to the withdrawal, but no one is really sure what is going on. Tests are being done tonight and in the morning. More information tomorrow. Brian's parents want to let everyone know that they appreciate their concern. However, during this very difficult time, they would like to remind everyone that they are requesting no visitors until further notice. Mom and Dad are not doing very well, and while well intentioned, having visitors at this time is more of a distraction to them and an interruption in Brian's recovery routine.*

8/23: Greeting day. Brian started going through periodic tremors yesterday that have continued into today. Last night, a CAT scan of his brain was ordered and the results came back normal. An electroencephalogram (EEG) was scheduled for early today, but that was cancelled. The care team explained that Brian's muscles and nerves want to move. It is still very scary to Mom and Dad. They have been allowed to start their visits earlier and stay later. Their presence seems to calm Brian down when he goes through these spells. The physical therapy team evaluated Brian today and will prepare a plan to start his treatment. The nurses and respiratory therapist continue to work on Brian's breathing. He is breathing on his own for part of the day, but still goes on the ventilator when sleeping. They also put the speaking valve on the trach this morning for practice. The care team tried to get Brian to say something, but he could not and it could take a few days for him to get used to the valve. When the ICU director made his morning rounds, he came into Brian's room and said, "Hello, everyone." Everyone looked at the ICU director, turning away from Brian, to say good morning. As all turned, Brian actually said, "Hello," through the valve. Everyone was stunned and turned around to face him. They cheered as he raised a shaky hand toward the ICU director. As doctor and patient shook hands, it became obvious that Brian has developed a connection with him.

8/24: Seven weeks today. Brian was given some medicine last night to help with the spells, so he was a bit groggy today. After his big day yesterday, the ICU director decided to let him rest today, and the respiratory therapist let him stay on the ventilator. When they did the morning patient assignment, the nurse who was selected to take care of Brian had never had him as a patient before. The other nurses looked at her and said that she better take good care of him because he was their baby. Mom and Dad saw two seizures today, a big one in the morning and a weaker one in the afternoon. These spells are *still frightening to them. Brian's nurse said he had a couple more, but not as many as yesterday. Brian's case manager gave them three rehab centers to evaluate. Even though this phase is going to be rough, it is what Mom and Dad have been waiting to hear, because it is a good sign. It shows that rehabilitation will be next. However, at the moment, Brian is so weak that he can barely lift a finger.*

To all Brian's friends: A hospital employee who has become a friend to Brian's parents is from Jamaica. She had her son, a Howard University student, bring back a Bob Marley T-shirt for Brian. She signed it, and hung it in Brian's room with a marker for everyone on the trauma team to sign. Oddly enough, Brian picked the family vacation this summer to celebrate his high school graduation. He chose Jamaica.

8/25: Slow day. The nurse called this morning and said Brian had only one episode through the night, at 5 a.m. He was a little more awake today because the ICU director stopped the heavy medication that makes him sluggish. The nurse let Mom and Dad stay a little longer to help wash his hair. He did have a few more episodes, one in the afternoon, one when Mom and Dad were leaving at night, and one more an hour later. Mom and Dad will need to be at the hospital early tomorrow because another feeding tube needs to be inserted.

8/26: Another slow day. However, Brian still had a few episodes. He is still working with his team, which includes a speech pathologist, an occupational therapist, and a physical therapist. No feeding tube surgery yet. With so many trauma cases coming into the hospital today, Brian's surgery kept getting delayed. They will not take him off the ventilator until he gets the feeding tube. Not much news today, but once again, no news is good news.

8/27: Kiss day. Mom and Dad toured one of the rehabilitation facilities this morning at 8 a.m. After their meeting, they arrived early at the hospital and the nurse said that they could go in to see Brian before visiting hours. As they walked into his room, his respiratory therapist was standing next to Brian while he was securely strapped into the hospital chair. She said that Brian had something for his mom, and she told him to show her. Brian slowly lifted his right arm, moving his hand slowly to his lips, and he blew her a kiss. Mom tried to keep the tears from showing because he was looking at her. She had to move behind his head as Dad kept things going so she could compose herself. They also received a smile with teeth showing. It was very faint, but he tried. Brian is waking up more and more each day, and this is very good. The hard part is that he is beginning to realize that he is in the hospital, cannot move well, and is hooked up to various machines. During the afternoon visit he woke up looking terrified, slowly moving his hand up to his neck, as he reached for the trach. The respiratory therapist tried to help comfort him. He is still having occasional seizures, but they seem to be less aggressive. It seems like the physical therapy, occupational therapy, and speech therapy, along with the visits from his parents, are making a difference. Mom and Dad have also been giving him face massages to try to get the muscles in his face used to moving again.

To all Brian's friends: Today was supposed to be Brian's "move in" day at his college. He was assigned to a dorm room with three roommates. Mom and Dad were thinking about this as they were visiting the rehab hospital. The other nice moment of the day, in addition to Brian's kiss and smile, was that his college swim coach called to check on him. He said when Brian is up to it, he and some of the guys would like to come and visit him. For all of you starting school on Monday, and to those already at college: do well, study hard, enjoy, and please think of Brian every now and then. He was so excited about going to college and swimming for the team. Mom and Dad tell him about his friends and family all over the world, and that he has new friends he does not even know yet.

8/28: Miracle day. The most wonderful day! Mom and Dad are too emotional after today's events to give their report. So many good things happened, they cannot even talk. All the details in tomorrow's update!

8/29: Amazing day, but first back to yesterday. Mom and Dad arrived for the morning visit, but had to call to get in. This was unusual. As the double doors opened, they saw a nurse who said, "You have to come see this." They almost broke into a run, but then saw the ICU director around the corner. Mom and Dad asked if everything was all right, and he answered, "I don't know," but did not look at them. He said, "You need to go in there." They looked at Brian's room and there were quite a few people in there. They walked in and heard, "Hi, Dad." Mom was behind Dad, but could not get to Brian because of the hugs and tears of joy from everyone. Brian then said, "Where's Mom?" She made it into the room, heard, "Hi, Mom," and then both Mom and Dad heard, "I love you guys." Brian continued to talk for two hours, thanking everyone in sight. He asked about all his friends, his grandparents and all the family, McDonough High School, and his college. He even asked, "How am I going to go to college or swim on the team?" Sad questions, but still a great sign that his brain is functioning. At one point, his dad was at a loss for words for the first time in two months. Brian looked at him and said, "Dad, it's OK. Everything is going to be all right." The nurses told Mom and Dad that when they put the speaking valve in, nobody expected him to talk. The ICU director was sitting outside Brian's room, and when he heard Brian talk, he shot out of his chair and ran into the room. The doctors and nurses are amazed at how he had woken up. They keep talking about the positive attitude he has. Then the three big questions: "What happened?", "Why am I here?", and "What's wrong with me?" Dad said he had been in a car accident and told him a few things, but then said, "We'll give you all the details when you're feeling better." Brian continued to talk, and talk, and talk. A good sign, because the nurse said that some people can handle the speaking valve for only fifteen minutes. Brian said he has been dreaming about a Mountain Dew Slurpee. The dietitian asked Brian what he would pick to eat when he passes the swallowing test, and she told his parents that it is usually a fast-food burger or a big steak. Brian told her, "Mandarin oranges or fruit cocktail." Everyone got a chuckle at that, because he is still Mr. Healthy. Then the radiology team came in to do a chest X-ray. As the nurse began explaining this to him, he looked at everyone and said, "It's OK. I've had lots of these, and I've had quite a few CAT scans too." Everyone just looked at each other, and nobody knew what to say. For the afternoon visit, the nurse left the speaking valve off because she had strict instructions not to let him get overtired. He did respond with his eyes and fingers, giving a thumbs-up to all questions. The other amazing thing today is that his body is moving: legs, right arm, neck, and face. However, the left arm is still extremely weak. The ICU director said that he is not taking any vacation, or even another day off until Brian goes to rehab. Mom and Dad went in for the night visit. As they walked in, the nurse told them to get a bottle of Mountain Dew. The ICU director said to give him a taste, even though the swallowing test would not be done until tomorrow. Mom and Dad brought in the soda and the nurse poured a tiny bit into a cup with a straw. She gave Brian a taste, and he said, "This is great."

Now back to today. Brian had his swallowing test, which determines not only whether he can eat, but also if the feeding tube in his nose can be removed. Everyone said it could take as many as three tries to pass this test. He was given the test with pudding, a milkshake, and then water, and he passed the first time. A lunch was delivered. He had Jell-O, grape juice, and banana pudding. He then continued to talk, and move his limbs a little bit. During the afternoon visit, Brian wrote with a pen and paper because he was resting from the speaking valve. Mom and Dad were allowed to stay most of the day, and the nurse put the speaking valve back in at four o'clock and it was still in when they left in the evening. The goal was to see if he could handle breathing on his own for twenty-four to forty-eight hours. When that happens, the trach can come out. His care team is taking it slow and trying to avoid any setbacks. Even Brian's trauma surgeon came by today. Brian shook his hand, thanked him, told him he really appreciated what he did, and said he loved him for saving his life. Words cannot even express the look of pure happiness on the faces of these doctors, physician assistants, nurses, and hospital employees. They say there is something very special about Brian. Honestly, from what Mom and Dad have seen, there is something very special about people in the medical profession, including the EMS providers—firefighters, rescue squads, and medevac crews.

8/30: Great day. Brian seemed worn out from all the excitement over the past few days, but he continued to talk. The speaking valve was put on at 7 a.m. and was still on when Mom and Dad left at night. The care team said they would probably take the valve off around 10 p.m. and put him back on the ventilator to let him sleep. He is now having trouble sleeping and looks extremely tired. They said it is almost like having jet lag. The director of nursing also explained to Brian that he has not returned to his natural sleep yet, but once he does, he will really sleep. He was chemically asleep for so long and this sleeping trouble is just another phase of the recovery. This is another reason they still discourage visitors. Due to the lack of sleep, he gets a bit emotional and frustrated. This can cause his breathing to fluctuate, and the goal continues to be weaning him off life support. The director of nursing also had a chat with Brian and told him she was in his shoes when she was twenty years old. Due to a medical problem, she had also been treated at this hospital and had been chemically induced. She knows exactly what he is going through. The ICU director requested that the case manager get the wheels rolling for Brian's rehab. Brian did eat today, but only a tiny bit. Everything is pureed. For lunch, he had a taste of turkey, veggies, mashed potatoes, apple juice, chocolate milk, and a chocolate-flavored vitamin-type drink. He did great. One of Brian's main doctors came by today to check on him. He is getting ready to leave for Jamaica, and the weird coincidence is that he is staying at the same resort where Brian and his parents stayed when they went in June. Brian talked to the doctor and thanked him for helping to save his life. He also told him that he looked buff, and asked if he played football. The doctor looked at him and said, "Yes, and I can't believe you didn't!"

8/31: Two months today. Brian continues to improve a little more. He ate each of his meals and was able to keep all of them down. He was switched from pureed food to slightly solid food. He continues to talk, but is still very tired because he has not yet reached his natural sleep. The ICU director explained that the ventilator is a contributing factor to his lack of restful sleep. He still goes on life support at night and the speaking valve comes out. He still has a positive attitude and continues to thank everyone in sight. He had so many doctors, physician assistants, nurses, and hospital staff in his room today that one of the other families' visitors asked if he was someone famous. There was good news today about his left arm too because of how weak it is. Brian was so worried that he asked his parents if he had to have his arm amputated. The physical therapist did a nerve test today, using electroshock. It was not pleasant, but results came back good. She said the nerves are bruised, but will come back over time with physical therapy. When Mom and Dad arrived this morning, he could raise his hand and forearm up to the elbow, but it is still a bit shaky. Brian continues to be anxious and scared about his health. The medical team believes this is caused by his lack of sleep, and that it is not a reason for concern. The doctors and nurses talk to him often to ease his fears, but he is starting to ask a lot of questions. For now, he still does not remember the accident, and hopefully he never will.

9/1: *Great day. Brian continues to improve. He is eating better, so the decision was made to take the feeding tube out of his nose. Brian promised everyone that he would try to eat more. He said he wants to get some strength back. He asked his nurse to hold his hand while the feeding tube was taken out. The care team spent a lot of time today moving him into different positions and explained that it is hard for Brian to get comfortable when he has been lying on his back for two months. The natural sleep may also be close because he is so exhausted.*

9/2: *Another great day. Guess who was on the phone this morning? The nurse called and put Brian on the phone to talk. When Mom and Dad arrived at the hospital in the morning, they were surprised to hear that Brian's trach would come out sometime today. The respiratory therapist walked into the room five minutes later and started laying out the gauze and tape. The care team proceeded to remove the trach. Dad stayed in the room while Mom stepped outside the closed curtain. Brian now has a gauze bandage over the opening left in his neck from where the trach used to be. It will close on its own in a few days. He is finally breathing 100 percent on his own, and the ventilator is no longer in the room. Brian has a long road ahead of him, but everyone says it is a true miracle.*

9/3: Another great day. Brian continues to improve more and more. His calorie intake is up to 1,800, but he needs to get to 3,000 per day. Brian said that he needs to put more meat on his bones. He stood up today with a walker and sat in a regular chair for fifteen minutes, but he got dizzy and was in agony. He promised his nurse that he would do better tomorrow.

9/4: Keeps on getting better. Brian continues to eat well, getting his calorie intake closer to what it should be. Once again, he had a bit of exercise, and did well, but it seriously tired him out. The doctors and nurses are extremely pleased with his progress.

9/5: Another day of healing. Brian spent some more time out of bed and in his hospital chair. He was able to stay in the chair for a longer period of time today. He is struggling somewhat with his appetite, but he is trying to get his calorie intake where it needs to be. There are happy and amazed expressions from some nurses and hospital personnel who are back on duty for the first time since Brian had his reawakening.

9/6: Super day! Brian is still coming along. He stood up on his feet today and took a few steps with the help of his nurse, Dad, and the walker. He is so skinny, he asked if the bones in his legs would break. It is heartbreaking to see the damage done to the body he had worked so hard to take care of. His physical therapist really motivated him hard today and it paid off with baby steps. She also said his mental attitude is great. Even the doctors and nurses said people do not usually wake up with this nice of a demeanor, but we all know Brian and how nice of a guy he is. He tried so hard with his therapy today that his nurse put him in a wheelchair to take a quick tour. She showed him around the trauma unit and even showed him the sci-fi bed he was in a few weeks ago. She then took him outside to get some fresh air. The look of life on his face was priceless.

9/7: Burger day. Brian did very well today. He was even more active, and to the pleasant surprise of all his doctors and nurses, continues to have a great attitude about his ongoing struggle to exercise his weakened muscles. We all know Brian and his work ethic, whether talking about academics or athletics, and we can only believe that he is going to come back stronger than ever. A bright spot for Brian after all his hard work today is that he earned a cheeseburger and fries as a little reward.

9/8: Another strong day. Brian continues to improve each day. He is more active, and the extra activity is less tiring for him. He is doing so well now that rehab will be coming soon. His appetite also continues to improve; calorie intake is up.

9/13: The best day ever. Brian is home! First, an explanation about the lack of updates. Everything happened so fast over the last five days. Last Tuesday, Brian was discharged from the ICU so he would be able to go to rehab. On Wednesday, he was taken by ambulance to a rehab center where he would start his therapy in five-day increments. His schedule began on Thursday with physical therapy two hours a day, then one hour of occupational therapy per day. His workouts have been tough because he could not stand or walk. He needs a wheelchair to get around. At this time, he is still very weak and is just skin and bones. Physical therapy was an amazing process to watch because he improved more and more each day. His weightlifting consisted of three pounds on his right arm and two pounds on the left arm, which is very hard for Brian to accept because he was a powerlifting champion during his junior year in high school. His rehab therapists explained that since Brian has been working so hard, he would be allowed to go home and continue his rehabilitation with outpatient physical therapy. At this time, Brian is still very limited. He cannot do anything on his own, and has to have his mom and dad around constantly to help him. His blood pressure has also been very high, and he is taking medication to treat this condition. Brian said he is not ready to see anyone just yet (he is still so very weak), but he hopes to be up for visitors very soon.

9/15: Highlight day. Brian's wheelchair was delivered today for him to use for the many trips to occupational therapy, physical therapy, and follow-up doctor visits that all begin next week. He is basically still bedridden and unable to walk or do anything on his own. He is extremely weak and physical therapy will probably last a long time. Mom and Dad ask him every day, but he is still not ready for visitors. He has tried to talk to his friends on the computer, but can last for only about fifteen minutes due to weakness. Also, telephone conversations seem to be too emotional for him right now, but he really appreciates the support from everyone.

9/16: Ambulance day. Not for Brian, but for his dad. This morning, Garth did not feel well and almost passed out; his symptoms included numbness, shortness of breath, and a heavy sensation on his chest. Mom called 911 and the volunteer rescue squad came to evaluate and transport him to the local hospital. When they came in, they went straight to Brian because he was the first one they saw. Dad was in the backyard, trying to get some air. On the way to the hospital, Dad told the EMT what has been happening with Brian, and she could not believe it because she said, "Is that the big, blond California kid that was in the accident with the dump truck?" It turns out she was one of the EMTs who had responded to the accident that day, and had actually been involved in helping Brian. Mom loaded up Brian and his wheelchair to go to the hospital. It took a while, but they eventually did get into the emergency room to see Dad. Mom and Brian ended up leaving the hospital because Brian was very uncomfortable and needed to go home.

His uncle came to stay with Dad and brought him home later that day. The hospital diagnosis was that Garth was suffering from hypertension and post-traumatic stress disorder (PTSD), which was brought on from everything he has been going through over the last few months. Mom, Dad, and Brian are all going to see the family doctor tomorrow. Maybe one day things will be normal again.

9/20: Healing weekend. Dad and Brian took it easy this weekend, trying to heal. A nurse called this morning from the ICU. All his wonderful doctors and nurses wanted to know how he is. They were actually surprised that he was already home from rehab. Brian still talks about all of them every day. Brian has a busy schedule this week with therapy starting tomorrow and several doctor follow-ups. Hopefully, all reports will be positive. The next update will be Friday after we get through all of the medical appointments.

9/27: Busy week. Brian started outpatient physical and occupational therapy, and it will continue for months. He is skin and bones, walks like he is ninety years old, and his blood pressure is still a concern. He went for follow-ups this week as well. When Brian and his parents walked in and saw Brian's trauma surgeon, they could sense that this man is very proud of what he does, and seeing Brian out of the hospital room is his reward. He told Brian's parents in the very beginning, "I love my patients," and the look in his eyes as he saw Brian just confirmed it. The trauma team has much to be proud of, even more than Brian's parents realized. Aside from all the physical trauma Brian sustained in the accident, the serious infections he later developed could have led to brain damage. The care he received was exceptional. Brian also saw his cardiologist from shock trauma. This was a big one for Mom and Dad because of the concern about all the initial damage to the heart. He did quite a bit of testing, including an EKG and echocardiogram. Mom and Dad nervously watched it all and finally got the great news. No fluid around the heart. The cardiologist was pleased with the results and, if all goes well, will not need to see Brian again for two years.

Brian's parents want to let everyone know that they are finally starting to get themselves together. This is truly another rough stage. In one respect, coming home with Brian is the ultimate relief. Words cannot express their joy, but it is still scary. They have no doctors or nurses around and one of them has to be with Brian at all times. He cannot do anything on his own. They literally watch him as he sleeps to see that he is breathing all right. When he takes a few steps, Mom has to hold him. They watch every move he makes. His medicine schedule is tricky and his sleeping pattern is out of sync. His body still seems to be on the schedule from the ICU, when the nurses would have to wake him every four hours to give him medicine, take his temperature, or perform blood work.

Luckily, Brian's parents seem to complement each other through this ordeal. Dad was not good in the beginning, mainly because of the original phone call he received about the accident and about Brian's condition. He was told that Brian was bleeding from the head and moving erratically, which would indicate head trauma. Why would a father be told this over the phone? That conversation stuck with Dad and, even though the tests came back saying there was no brain damage, he had to wait two months to really believe it. Mom fell apart during the middle of the hospital stay, and then again in the rehab hospital, which was not an easy experience for any of them. It is no surprise that, since Dad carried the brunt of it all, he ended up in the hospital when he came home.

It has been a very difficult adjustment going from twenty-four-hour-a-day care by the wonderful staff at the ICU to handling all of Brian's day-to-day needs by themselves with no additional support. As frightening as the hospital stay was and as low as the lows could be, the highs for Brian's parents were amazingly high. To have a child survive such a horrific accident, and then recover as Brian has, certainly takes an incredible emotional toll. The roller coaster has come to an abrupt halt, and along with it, the adrenaline level as well.

Now, Brian and his parents have to deal with the incredibly difficult task of physical therapy. What keeps everyone going is Brian. His attitude is outstanding, almost unbelievable. He does have a weak moment every so often. He watches his track and swim tapes, but does not feel sorry for himself, and says he will be back. As feeble and scarred as he is, he took baby steps past the mirror today and posed as if he had his muscles. It was actually a sad sight to watch. He made the comment that his abs are coming back, but it is actually because he is so skinny. It was said again by his doctors this week that he is a true miracle.

***10/5**: Therapy week. Brian continues with physical and occupational therapy. In PT, they had him try Tai Chi this week. He has a hard time with this because it is a slow-paced and peaceful workout program, which is something Brian is not used to, but it is all he can do for now. In OT, they are using E-Stim on his left arm. E-Stim is a treatment that sends an electronic stimulus directly into the muscle tissue. The feeling it gives is like pins and needles. Brian is tempted to get back in the pool, but must wait until his blood pressure gets under control. Since he is still in a wheelchair, he also needs to improve his standing and walking.*

***10/19**: Up-and-down couple of weeks—sorry for the delay. Brian's parents are still not with it. They have not forgotten any of you and what everyone has done for them and Brian. They will call, write, visit, etc. as soon as they get it together—promise. The week of the twelfth, Brian started to get a cold,* *which created fear again for his parents, but they got it under control. He continued with OT and PT. There was another scare last week because his blood pressure went up again. Trying to wean him off the medicine may take some time. His blood pressure shot up to 151/101 when he went one day without the pill. Plus, that interfered with his OT and PT because each therapist had to have him rest. Since Brian woke up, it has been like having a baby because he is learning to do everything again. He is very self-conscious of his condition, and it is because of this that he still has not really seen any of his friends, except when Brian's parents took him for a ride and stopped by a popular coffee shop near where they live. Three of his good friends were inside the shop when Mom walked in. She told them Brian was outside with Dad in the truck. They ran out to see him and were so excited; they could not believe how skinny he was. Brian was glad to see them, but he still continues to hold off on having visitors until he gets more mobile and some weight back. He has some good friends here and some who will be coming home from different colleges in the next few weeks, so hopefully, he will be ready to see them all. His parents are beginning to think that would be good for him. The ICU director was so right when he kept telling them, "If Brian makes it through this, it will be a long road." They now know what he meant. With a little help from all of you, all over the world, through the power of your prayers, Brian is recovering. You are part of the miracle.*

Suggestions for Health Care Providers and/or Patient's Family:

- The health care providers see families that are dealing with grief on a daily basis, but a new family that is just entering the hospital with a loved one has no idea what to expect. These families are often put in positions where they have to continuously report the patient's health status to every friend and family member who comes to visit or calls on the phone. Not every patient will be fortunate enough to have a lot of people coming to visit. It is heartwarming to see such an outpouring of generous support, but having to repeat the information over and over can take a heavy toll on the mind and body. The care provider can recommend a strategy, like providing daily health status updates on a website, so families do not have to keep repeating the same traumatic information.

- Since technology is advancing by the minute, there are a lot of new electronic communication sites that exist today. The hospital could provide informational links to families or friends on how to establish a site to report their loved one's condition. The hospital could even include these details on its own website and the care providers could suggest to loved ones that they go there to find details on what websites they can choose from.

- In most cases, the people closest to the patient (parents, husband, wife, significant other, etc.) have an incredible workload just trying to take care of the patient. It might be helpful for the care provider to help the family designate a spokesperson to share news and updates on the status of the patient (via text message, phone calls, emails, and a website) so those closest to the patient will not have to worry about trying to keep others informed.

- There are many benefits to maintaining a website, especially one that has a format where people can write messages and thoughtful notes of inspiration. These encouraging messages not only help motivate everyone who has permission to view the website, but also bring strength to the closest members of the family who are looking after the patient every day. These messages can have a very motivational influence on the patient when, and if, he or she is able to view them.

Reflective Questions for Health Care Providers (write your answers in Part Five):

1) Do you personally believe that keeping a daily health status website can be beneficial for the patient's family? Under what circumstances? Explain why you feel that way.

2) When you know that a patient is going to be long term, do you recommend to his or her family that it might be helpful for them to look into creating a website that will give a daily update on the patient's health status?

3) If you do recommend a website to the family that will provide daily health updates, which one do you recommend the most? Why?

4) Can you remember a specific time that you heard about the benefits of using the website?

5) How should hospital personnel relate the news of an accident on the phone? How can the patient's serious condition be relayed without causing too much alarm or stress?

PART TWO

CARE

"You must never so much think as whether you like it or not, whether it is bearable or not; you must never think of anything except the need, and how to meet it."

—Clara Barton

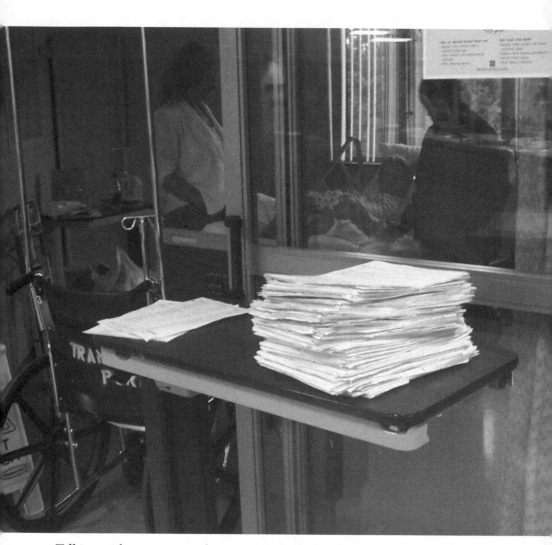

Talking with my mom and a nurse in the hospital room. My stack of medical records is sitting on the small table outside the room.

CHAPTER 4

PATIENT- AND FAMILY-CENTERED CARE

During each revolving shift, the care providers and the patient's family are striving toward progress. They want these men, women, and children to heal, and their actions are enabling any potential improvements. The patient may be only one person, but in the big picture, the path to progress is never an individual effort.

Former patients and their families can influence improvements in patient care by partnering with health care providers in advisory groups. The patient and family members share their personal accounts of their time in the hospital, which help health care staff see those experiences from a different vantage point so they can address overall patient satisfaction, quality of care, and safety concerns (Warren, 2012).

The Institute for Patient- and Family-Centered Care (2010) defines the concept of patient- and family-centered care as, "An approach to the planning, delivery, and evaluation of health care that is grounded in mutually beneficial partnerships among health care providers, patients, and families." This multi-disciplinary approach includes the family in the decision-making process with the care team. Not only do the families get to participate by listening to the care team discuss their treatment plan, but the families will also be able to provide valuable insight and feed-back regarding the upcoming procedures. Sacco, Stapleton, and Ingersoll (2009) found that family support groups co-facilitated by the families of former ICU patients can bring forth important care delivery issues that might not be mentioned in sessions that are only initiated by the care providers.

Similar to a mechanical system of interlocked gears, the communica-tion among the patient, family, and health care providers is very impor-tant throughout the entire recovery process.

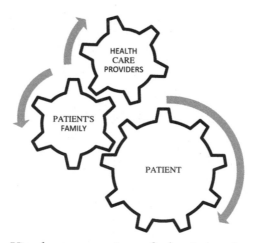

Visual representation of the interaction among the patient, patient's family, and health care providers.

Assuming that a healthy and stable relationship exists, the family knows the patient better than anyone else in the world because they have spent years living with or in close proximity with this person. In the hos-pital, you can spend a few minutes or even a few hours with a patient in order to get to know his or her likes and dislikes, as well as a brief under-standing of his or her background. However, no matter how much time you spend with a patient, the family, especially the parents, will have the advantage when it comes to knowing the patient best. The maternal and paternal bonds develop when their child is born, and this genetically acquired connection is so powerful that they are able to recognize practically imperceptible physical and behavioral changes when nobody else can. The family and friends will typically know the common gestures, movements, body language, personality traits, inner thoughts, idiosyncrasies, behaviors, and typical phrases and concerns of their loved one.

On numerous occasions when I have talked to parents about their children who were unconscious, comatose, or in a catatonic state, they discussed with me how they were aware of the feelings and emotions of their children—even though no words were spoken. The patient's body may appear almost lifeless to anybody else in the room, but to the parents there is almost a telepathic interaction that takes place where they can see visible signs of life. Their level of awareness originates from their love, which is unbounded by the normal limits of science and medicine.

Familial instincts proved very important on a few occasions with my parents, especially on one particular day. When they arrived for a visit, they noticed that it sounded like my chest was congested and that my trach secretions in the container next to my bed seemed quite thick. My parents asked the respiratory therapist about the sounds of congestion, but he said that he had just suctioned my trach. Mom and Dad are not medical people, but they did not have a good feeling about it for some reason. They remained in my room, quietly watching me breathe and watching over the tubes and wires connected to me. As the visiting hour ended, they went down to the lobby to sit until they could return for their next visit a few hours later.

The next visit did not happen as planned. As they sat waiting, my mom received a phone call on her cell phone from the ICU requesting that they return to the unit immediately. My parents sprinted through the long halls to get to my room, all the while knowing that something really bad must have happened. Truthfully, they thought I passed away.

As the big steel doors slammed open, they ran into the unit and saw a lot of people standing over me in my room, which was quite disheveled. Their faces looked stressed, and all eyes were on me in the hospital bed. My parents looked in my room and saw that I was lying there with the blue intubation tube back in my mouth. It was an eerie sight because my body was lying completely flat on the bed. The pillows had been thrown off the bed and the bed linens were scattered. The hospital room sort of resembled the look of a morgue.

My mom immediately broke down. The doctors and nurses reassured my parents that I was alive and the intubation had worked. They had to perform an emergency intubation because I was in a dire situation. A nurse was walking by my room and noticed that my face was turning blue, which meant oxygen was not flowing through my trach tube, most likely due to a clog. The nurse hit the code button to alert that she needed immediate assistance. Everyone raced into my room, saw that I was not breathing, and I was quickly intubated. I was then taken to surgery to have a new tracheostomy tube placed in my neck, and my lungs vacuumed out.

At that time, nobody really knew if there had been a loss of oxygen to my brain. We had come so far in the recovery process, but this one incident could have been fatal. My parents had a gut instinct that something was not right when they were visiting with me earlier that day. Their intuition that something was wrong proved accurate. This particular incident validates how important it is to include the observations and feedback from the family when treating the patient.

WHEN YOU ARE FOCUSING ON THE GOALS FOR THE PATIENT'S RECOVERY, the doctors work with the nurses, specialists, and patient's family to decide on the appropriate care plan for the patient on both a short- and long-term basis. It is vital that this multi-disciplinary approach occurs during the formation of the care plan and is frequently updated as time goes on.

A helpful way to illustrate the contributions of these groups into the care plan is to look at the 4x100 relay event in track and field. You have four runners who will each run a total of 100 meters, which will result in one complete lap (400 meters in length). The runners are located at designated areas on the track, and the first runner will carry the baton to the second runner, followed by the third, and the fourth runner will carry the baton to the finish line. Each runner equally contributes his or her time, energy, and experience to go from point A (starting line) to point B (finish line). The nurses, doctors, specialists, and family members are working with the patient and contributing their time, energy, and observations into getting the patient from point A (sick patient) to point B (healthy patient). These groups in the care team should do their best to contribute their expertise and align their strategies to form the most effective plan of treatment where equality is emphasized.

Each group spends time observing the patient; therefore each can contribute to the overall treatment plan. Still, I remember noticing that there was an occasional disconnect between some groups of care providers. There is absolutely no time to compare resumes, degrees, and CVs when the patient's life is on the line. There should not be any hierarchical discrepancies in the health care system, and egos should be left out entirely. Each group is formally trained in its own disciplines, and the educated feedback from each group can potentially provide a missing link that could ultimately lead to a breakthrough in the patient's recovery. The family may not have a medical degree, nursing license, or doctorate, but their observations can be very effective.

Dr. Peter Pronovost, in his innovative book *Safe Patients, Smart Hospitals*, describes how the care plan is the most effective when each group collaborates in the decision-making process. "Each of the members of a patient's team, including a parent if the patient is a child, sees problems through a different set of lenses that is shaped by personal experiences and training. Each of those lenses provides valuable information."

Each group spends time observing the patient, therefore every group can contribute to the overall treatment plan. There are so many advantages to taking this approach, because every voice is heard, every concern is addressed, and every potential approach is analyzed by the overall team before a plan is pursued. This plan is truly enriched because all contributing groups provide their input, helping to get the patient from his or her current state of being sick or injured to the finish line of his or her recovery.

Suggestions for Health Care Providers and/or Patient's Family:

- If there is no support group, perhaps a Point of Contact could be available for information or questions. Doctors and nurses are extremely busy and not always available.
- A hospital information guide for visitors (Appendix) would be helpful. This guide would provide hospital phone numbers, visiting hours, parking and cafeteria information, nearby hotel listings, and simple medical-term definitions. It would also be helpful to include details on what family members should expect or be required to do, including behavior. My parents saw so

many rude families who had loved ones inside the unit treating the medical people badly, even to the point of trashing the waiting room. Everyone reacts to grief differently, but to take it out on the doctors and nurses trying to save lives is just not right.

• Listen to the feedback from the people who know the patient best (parents, family, significant others, and close friends) because they may notice a small lifesaving detail in the patient that the care providers are unable to see.

Reflective Questions for Health Care Providers (write your answers in Part Five):

1) Do you feel that you always try to engage with the patient? Please explain in more detail.

2) Do you feel that you always try to engage with the patient's family? Please explain in more detail.

3) Are there any circumstances that would keep you from engaging with a patient or his or her family?

4) When you have a new patient and you meet his or her family for the first time, are there certain things that you do that help put them at ease?

5) Do you listen and engage with the patient's family and close friends to help the way that you treat the patient?

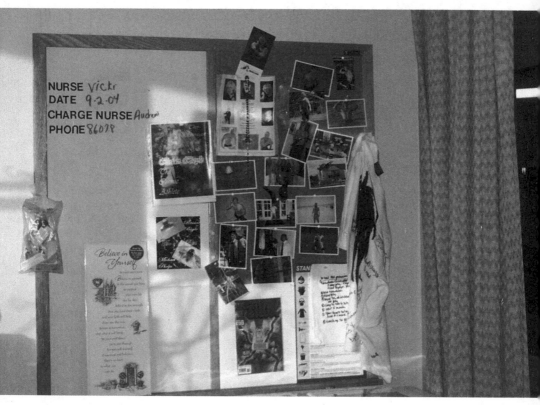

The view of the bulletin board in my hospital room.

CHAPTER 5

SENSATION AND PERCEPTION

I REGAINED CONSCIOUSNESS IN A HOSPITAL BED WITH NO MEMORY OF what had happened to me, where I was, and what was going to happen in the future. My initial thoughts revolved around a few major questions. Why was I paralyzed? Why was I unable to talk? Why could I see only a portion of the room? Why were my parents crying every time I saw them? What was the reason behind all this suffering? Would it be like this for the rest of my life? Every day there were new questions, but no answers.

My vision was dependent on whatever angle I was lying at in the hospital bed, and my sense of touch was affected by the heavy sedation. I could not talk, move, or reliably follow any commands, but my sense of hearing was hypersensitive. I was very aware of my surroundings as a result of my sensitivity to sound, the only sense available to me.

My mind was relentlessly craving any type of sensation or stimulation. On the surface I was not experiencing much physical pain because of the powerful effects of the morphine and other paralyzing painkillers, but the mental anguish of being trapped in this physical prison was extremely frustrating.

Maniou (2012) explained that "patients are simultaneously subjected to a threat to life, the awe of medical procedures, an inability to communicate needs, a new and threatening environment, and the loss of personal control." As I lay in a hospital bed, day in and day out, hour after hour, it became physically exhausting and highly taxing on the mind.

Intensive care unit (ICU) delirium occurs in 20 percent to 80 percent of patients (Desai, Chau & George, 2013). The potential for ICU delirium can be managed through maintaining the safe environment, educating on ICU delirium, communicating with patients and relatives frequently and effectively, improving sleep quality, and controlling the situation (Fan, Guo & Zhu, 2012).

The only way that I could temporarily escape my situation was by shutting my eyes, but most of the time my eyes were frozen open and I was too weak to close them. They would put Lacri-Lube drops in my eyes to keep them from drying out, but this would blur my vision almost entirely. I did not want to close my eyes anyway, because I had been asleep already for a few weeks and I depended on my vision and hearing to make sense of what was going on around me. I needed answers, and I needed to remain on constant alert.

I was highly tuned in to this unfamiliar environment. Whether I was in my hospital room, or being taken to get an operation, CAT scan, or one of the several dozen X-rays, I was observing anything and everything that happened around me. I was aware of the people, conversations, places, locations, and glimpses of the walls or bulletin boards. These fragmented pieces of information were like a jigsaw puzzle of reality.

I felt like a lone traveler who had washed up on a deserted island and had to devote every ounce of energy to being saved. My main problem was that I was paralyzed, immobile, and had to rely heavily on my eyes and ears to obtain information on my surroundings and plan my rescue.

It was an ongoing battle to keep my mind from going over the edge. Instead of focusing on things that I had no control over, I switched my thought process over to seeking temporary distractions and interpreting the stimuli around me for the answers to all of my questions and concerns.

Mind Games

It became an ongoing search for pain-relieving distractions—anything that would help me momentarily escape the lonely life that I was leading on the hospital bed. I would try my best to occupy my mind with games that I could play from my horizontal, static position. It was a simple method to waste time, but these games also served as a therapeutic outlet that allowed me to maintain my sanity.

I had the perfect view of the ceiling, which was covered in the standard off-white speckled insulated tile that you typically see in hospitals. I would count the small holes in each tile frame, and then move onto the next tile, and then the next. It was not a rare occurrence when I found myself counting up to the thousands, or even the tens of thousands. I had all the time in the world to do this and the fact that it was mind numbing made it even more useful.

When I could not count any further, or I accidentally lost my position on the tile, I would watch the light softly flicker in the lightbulbs and would almost fall into a trance. I do not know if it was a combination of being in this trance or the sedation I was on, but I would hallucinate by staring at a fixed point for a few minutes. Before I knew it, I felt released from my stationary position. The restraints vanished and I fought gravity millimeter by millimeter as I raised myself to an upright position, immediately feeling the weight of the world on my weakened shoulders. I softly placed my bare feet on the cold floor, feeling so emaciated that I could barely raise myself forward. I would then slowly sneak out of the hospital room and the ICU, where freedom awaited me at each new step.

In my trance-like state, I was free to move around to anywhere I wanted to venture for minutes or even hours, if my mind would allow it. No matter how far I traveled, my final destination would always be back to my hospital bed. I had no choice but to return my focus to physically healing, because my imagination was not going to be the only factor in helping me leave the hospital room. My mind was active and strong, but unfortunately my body was not.

Mouth Care

My mouth was dry and my tongue felt like a shriveled-up piece of sandpaper that had been scraped all the way down to a fine sheet. I constantly fantasized about having something nice and cool to quench my thirst, and not a minute would go by without my mind fixing on this craving.

There was a round analog clock above my hospital room doorway that was similar to the style from my primary school years, with the hour, minute, and second hands slowly rotating around the center dial. It seemed like my life stopped the first moment I was brought into the hospital, but this clock was proof that the outside world was not waiting for me to get better. It was a distinct reminder that life was advancing right outside my room, and it was up to me to get back into it. I became fixated on the clock.

I used the clock as a form of distraction. I would watch the second hand slowly tick by, and every fifteen seconds I would tease my imagination with the thought of drinking a tall glass of ice water. Fifteen more seconds would pass, and the fantasy switched over to apple juice, and then Mountain Dew. It was not uncommon to daydream for an entire minute about chugging a gallon container of lemon-lime Gatorade. This was a rare treat, and I savored every second of it.

Any time that someone from my care team came into my room and interacted with me, he or she would immediately wash his or her hands in the sink on the left side of my room. I looked forward to the moment when he or she turned on the water faucet and I became captivated by the trickle of liquid just a few feet away from me.

Sometimes, during a sponge bath when the nurses would be washing my hair, I fantasized that I might be fortunate enough to have a tiny splash of water land in my dry desert of a mouth. There was one time where I remember my wish coming true, and it brought instant relief.

For these reasons aforementioned, routine mouth care is very important to do every few hours. In normal circumstances, people get thirsty and they need something to drink. Until that need is met, the sensation of thirst increases until satisfied. As a ventilated (initially intubated and then trached) and nothing-by-mouth (NPO) patient, I was given IV fluids and nasogastric feeds, which met my metabolic needs. However, I still experienced thirst and it was always on my mind.

It made such an impact when small measures of mouth care were carried out during my daily treatment. I longed for my teeth to be cleaned, because that would allow moisture to be in my mouth, even for just a very short time. I gradually understood why I could not be given any fluids by mouth, but it would have relieved so much suffering if my team could have put a small wet sponge or damp swab in my mouth just to appease that nagging sensation of always being extremely parched.

As my recovery progressed, and my body was being weaned off the sedation, my strength slowly came back, and I learned how to talk again. I could communicate for short periods of time and easily follow commands. It would have been satisfying (and efficient) to take a sip of water, swish it around my mouth, and then have it suctioned out.

Spiritual Needs

My faith has always been very important to me and it played a large role throughout my recovery. In times when I was having difficulty in understanding why things happened the way they did, my beliefs helped me step back and look at the big picture in order to find meaning and an overall sense of inner peace. I may have been on life support and hooked up to many lifesaving machines, but I was still on this earth. I was still alive.

An individual's religion is a very personal component of his or her identity and his or her outlook on life. Faith can provide hope and comfort along the path to recovery. The appropriate measures should be taken to educate the patient and family of what services are available, what arrangements can be made, if there are any designated areas in the hospital that they can go to, and if any significant religious items can be placed in the hospital room to comfort the patient. I encourage care providers to accommodate the spiritual needs of the patient and family, because I truly feel that it can aid in the healing process.

Reiki

Reiki is a Japanese healing technique that reduces stress and promotes relaxation. I first learned about it at a nursing conference where they discussed the benefits of using Reiki in a hospital setting. According to the International Center for Reiki Training (2014), Reiki feels like a wonderful glowing radiance that flows through and around your body, working in conjunction with all other medical or therapeutic techniques to relieve side effects and promote recovery. The more I learned about this technique, the more I realized how effective it could be for certain patients because it would engage their senses and energy. In their book, *Reiki Energy Medicine: Bringing Healing Touch into Home, Hospital, and Hospice*, Libby Barnett and Maggie Chambers discuss how Reiki can be effective in hospital settings because, "It helps relieve stress, agitation, and acute or chronic pain; it is helpful as an aid for sleeping and also as an energizer. It promotes the release of emotions such as grief, anger, or anxiety and provides comfort in palliative care." Perhaps it would have been helpful for the caregivers to try practicing Reiki with me while I was healing.

Visual and Audio

When things were pretty calm in my hospital room and I was alone, I would try to hear what was taking place within the rest of the ICU. This was a difficult task, because the electronic beeps and mechanical blips from my lifesaving medical equipment continuously filled the air. Underneath these sounds there was always a gentle humming noise near my bed that sounded like an air conditioner, but it was actually part of my ventilator. The peaceful sound of silence never truly existed. Despite the cacophony, I managed to find a way to rest.

Throughout the day I would hear pages on the intercom made up of coded medical messages being relayed to specialized teams within the unit and throughout the rest of the hospital, especially when it involved incoming shock trauma patients.

There was a red alarm on the outside of every room near the top of the doorframe. When this alarm went off, a siren would begin blaring and a red light would flash to signal that the patient in that room needed assistance. A select group of nurses and doctors on shift scrambled to that room to help stabilize the patient.

On more than one occasion, when my medical equipment reported that my body was failing, the electronic beeps would gradually increase in frequency and volume. Before I knew it, the alarm outside my room would be sounding off, and several people would rush into my room. They quickly read the vitals, looked at the medical equipment, found the part of my body that was in trouble, and either took me to the radiology department or the operating room. It was a frightening ordeal when this occurred, but I knew I was in good hands with these amazing people.

THERE WAS A TELEVISION IN THE UPPER RIGHT CORNER OF MY ROOM, AND it was always a treat when it was tuned to a channel that had a program I enjoyed watching. My care team knew about my athletic background in swimming and running, because they talked with my parents about this regularly and they saw the photos of my teammates and me on the bulletin board in my room. It provided so much rejuvenation to my body, mind, and spirit when they turned the TV on so I could watch events that I loved.

The volume from the television came from a remote control that was hooked up to my bed, and depending on the shift and the nurse whom I had, he or she would usually put the remote next to my shoulder so I could hear the broadcasted programs. This proved tricky, as sometimes the volume was too loud because the remote was so close to my head and I was not able to communicate to lower the sound level.

Before the accident, I did not watch TV that often. However, as a patient in the hospital I did everything in my power to visually show my nurses that I enjoyed having the television on. Through a twitch of the finger or a gentle flutter of my eye, I was able to communicate this to them on a more reliable basis as each week went by.

I understand that medical treatment and patient observations are always top priority. However, when everything is thoroughly accounted for, it's nice to consider the patient's enjoyment of television as well. If the patient shows any visible interest in watching television, you could assist the patient and select programs that are wholesome and positive. Scary movies and horror films can be quickly skipped over until an alternative selection is available.

Television is best enjoyed by patients anytime from the morning through the evening, and should be switched off at night to allow the patient to rest. If the patient becomes agitated when the television is on during the day, or is not engaged with the screen, then it should be immediately turned off. If the patient is unable to show interest or is unresponsive, I personally would recommend having the TV on just in case.

In my situation, I was both medically paralyzed and unresponsive, and having the TV on worked wonders for my overall morale. My favorite program was the Olympics, and I did not mind watching the local news, a random movie that may have been on, or even the station where they played relaxing music with a steady slideshow of scenic photos. It would get even more exciting if they showed any type of beverages in these shows, or an advertisement for water, juice, or soda.

The television provided an outlet for escape that was a thousand times greater than staring at the dots on ceiling tiles or the flicker of electricity bouncing around in the fluorescent lightbulbs. Instead of having to day-dream about quenching refreshments while looking at the clock in my room, I could see the real thing on TV, which was almost as satisfying.

At this time of my recovery I was still paralyzed on heavy sedation and my response to commands was not always reliable. Even though I could not respond or show satisfaction in my face when they turned the TV on, I was smiling from ear to ear beneath my frozen disposition.

Music

Music has the ability to instantly distract us from our suffering and pain, letting us focus on something hopeful instead (Briggs, 2011). You can be at one of the lowest moments in your life, and when you turn on your favorite song you can be on top of the world. If there is one place where the healing power of music should thrive, it is in the hospital room.

In an excellent book titled *The Sounds of Healing*, Dr. Mitchell Gaynor describes the recuperative power of music when he states that, "We accept that sound is vibration, and we know that vibration touches every part of our physical being, then we understand that sound is 'heard' not only through our ears but through every cell in our body."

The initial weeks of living in hospital room 19 consisted of multiple lifesaving operations and high-anxiety procedures that required constant supervision and reevaluation. It was near the end of the first month when it became evident that my treatment would be long term. Would I remain in the ICU for a few more weeks, or would I be transferred to a nursing home?

It was a waiting game and the duration of time that I would remain in the ICU was completely unknown. Even though I was coherent, people were unsure of my level of comprehension, and I had no direct control over the actual progress and physical setbacks with my recovery. My mind and body felt like two disconnected components. It was up to me to secure that vital connection to continue on with the recovery, but it was slow and tedious work.

It was around this time that one of my main nurses suggested to my parents that it would be therapeutic if they brought in a CD player to play music for me. My parents liked her idea, and the next day they walked into the room proudly holding a little stereo system the size of a basketball and carrying some of my favorite CDs. I was ecstatic when I saw that they were going to play music for me.

There were four CDs per sheet, and my dad would lift the binder up in the air and carefully point to each one as he read the musician and album title. I knew the names and precise locations of the CDs in the binder, so this method not only helped me, but also was a way for my parents and care providers to observe how I was visually interacting with their questions. They would watch my eyes as I focused in on each sheet, which was a big deal because it showed that I was engaged with what they were doing.

I would attentively blink my eyes when my dad mentioned a musician or band that I was interested in. As soon as he mentioned my favorite band, I quickly shut my eyes and reopened them. To confirm this was the right choice, my dad would ask me again and I would follow up with the same response.

When my mom placed the CD in the stereo, I was transported to a happier time and place. A world without machines breathing for me, without sadness, and without all those obstacles in my way. In that moment, I was just a regular young guy listening to his favorite band.

From the first time my mom turned on the little stereo in my room, it stayed on. When a CD was not on, my dad would make sure that a favorite radio station of mine was playing in the background.

The ICU was still a very serious place, with critically ill patients clinging to life as I was, but when the music was playing in my hospital room, it changed everything for me. Suddenly I was free. There was a light at the end of the tunnel; there was warmth from sunshine, and there was color back in my monochromatic world. With that said, music should always be kept at an appropriate volume in the hospital room to prevent any potential distractions to the care providers; the sounds of the medical equipment should still be clearly audible over the music. Similar to the TV, the radio or music player should be switched off at night to allow the patient to rest.

My care team would also alternate between the TV and radio, which I enjoyed because it provided a variety of stimulation for my senses. My parents tried their best to find the type of music that I liked, but they also made sure that it would be something that was calm and soothing. Music that consists of soft sounds has the potential to significantly reduce stress and pain with patients being treated in intensive care (Trappe, 2012).

The potential for music to create a positive impact in a patient's progress cannot be underestimated and should be included in his or her daily routine. As Bob Marley said, "One good thing about music, when it hits you, you feel no pain."

Bulletin Board

There was a large bulletin board on the wall in my room. It was a standard white dry erase board, and the name of my nurse, the date, the name of my charge nurse, and my room's phone number was always written on it. Since I was completely dependent on external information to understand my situation, it would have been nice to include a few more things on this bulletin board that pertained to my setting and sense of motivation.

When posting on the bulletin board, the most important thing is to make sure that medical information takes precedence. As a patient, I was glad to see the name of the nurse who was taking care of me, as well as the charge nurse for that designated time. I had so many care providers looking after me throughout each shift, and I paid attention to what their names were because it was a comfort to be able to put names to the faces of the people looking after me. Even when I was unable to talk, it was nice to know their names because I could keep track of these small details.

When I started to become a little more aware of my surroundings, I was not quite sure what day of the week it was, or the month, or even the year. I was not even sure how old I was when I woke up, which was frightening. In order to understand the duration of time and connect the dots, I had to venture back into that time frame after I was released from the hospital and consult with my parents and care providers based on the earliest memories that I had upon waking up. It helped that they included the date on the bulletin board, but because I was not aware of how long I had been in the hospital, it would have been helpful to include the total number of days that I had been a patient too. My grasp of time would have improved greatly, especially if this number was updated daily.

I have always liked setting goals, both in the long and short terms, because it gives me something to strive for. After the accident, everything changed. All the goals I had planned for myself were drastically altered, my path was diverted into the unknown, and I was not sure that I would ever be able to pursue them again. In the meantime, it would have helped me regain some of the much-needed control in my life if my care team posted one or two goals that were expected of me at that point of my recovery.

For example, "The goal for today is to respond with blinking eyes, moving fingers, or wiggling toes." Seeing this on the bulletin board not only would have motivated me, but would have provided me an adequate amount of time to prepare for accomplishing these goals. The atmosphere in the hospital is very fast-paced, and listing these goals would be an effective way to slow the pace down and direct the patient's attention to a few specific details. When a goal is achieved, you move onto the next one. Over time, short-term goals are transformed into long-term goals, a sense of stability is slowly returned to the patient, and progress continues along this new path.

Another supplemental boost of motivation would be an inspirational quote, or a message written by a loved one. Similar to signing a friend's yearbook or writing encouraging words on a friend's cast, the motivational message will be a part of the patient's comfort zone. When looking at these messages, the patient will have a constant reminder that he or she is not going through this alone and that there is a team of people supporting the patient as he or she gets better.

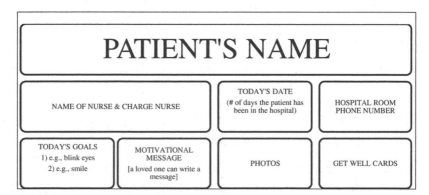

Sample of visual layout of patient's bulletin board.

Motivational Items

As the weeks went by, I noticed an increasing number of get well cards that surrounded the bulletin board in my room. I received letters from family, friends, and even strangers who were supporting my recovery. From my hometown, to all the way around the world, it meant a lot to me that people were taking the time to write these letters to let me know they were thinking of me and hoping that my recovery continued. Sometimes my parents or care providers would read the letters to me or let me know who had written to me. I did not mind that they read my cards, and when I was able to talk again, I encouraged them to read the cards because it was a way that my care team could get to know me a little better.

Dr. Katrina Firlik, a neurosurgeon, discusses her experiences and background in the book *Another Day in the Frontal Lobe*. When talking about get well cards in a patient's room, she explains that, "Those are the things that make me feel like I kind of know the person lying in the bed, unconscious, whom I have never truly met, and may never get to meet."

My nurses also encouraged my parents to bring pictures that personified my life so they could get to know me. They posted the photos on a section of the bulletin board that documented my life before the accident. There were photos of me participating in my favorite sports, like swimming and track and field, playing guitar, enjoying summer vacation with my parents, and hanging out with friends and family. Seeing these photos made a positive impact on me because I was able to reflect on a lot of great memories. As sterile and intimidating as my hospital room was from all the lifesaving equipment, these mementos helped transform my current world into "my room." There was an atmosphere of comfort having these images within my new home away from home.

I was proud of the life I had lived before the accident, and in the same way that I encouraged my care team to look at my get well cards, I also requested that they look at the photos. You feel very vulnerable as a patient, practically naked to the world in a thin hospital gown. Modesty does not exist in the hospital room, especially in the ICU, and when you really look at the big picture, you are ultimately just a body. However, I wanted to project myself as something more than just skin, bones, and an extensive array of injuries and scars. Maybe it was because I felt very self-conscious, but in my mind, these photos were proof that I was a person with a past, a life, a family, and a future.

As an athlete for most of my life, my health and fitness were very important to me and I always tried to stay in good shape. Even though my new body was scarred and slightly cadaverous in appearance, it was nice to have photos that showed my visitors and care providers that I did not always look like this. These photos were also a great conversation starter for my care team because they would occasionally walk over to the bulletin board, look at the photos, look at me on the hospital bed, and an interaction would take place.

My family and friends brought a variety of gifts that were placed in a designated area near the bulletin board: stuffed animals with get well messages on them, *Thor* comic books, T-shirts, swim goggles, a rosary, an inspirational poster, and various drawings and artwork that my loved ones made for me. When you introduce such items to a patient's room, they may bear a lot of significance for the patient.

Stress-Relief Ball

My parents brought in a small foam stress-relief ball that was green and blue and resembled the Earth. My dad told me that the world was now in the palm of my hands as he gently wrapped my fingers around it. Both he and my mom told me to squeeze this ball whenever I could, which was close to impossible when they first gave it to me. At the time, I was still heavily sedated and my ability to physically respond to commands was extremely limited. Even with my faint strength, I tried my best to squeeze the foam ball, but it barely amounted to any more than a slight tremble of my hand. I remained persistent.

From the initial phase of just twitching my fingers around the ball, it progressed after a few weeks to being able to squeeze the entire ball, which was assisted by the fact that I was slowly being weaned off the heavy medication. Sometimes throughout the daily activity and various procedures, the ball would fall out of my hand, but it would be returned to me within an hour or two and I would continue my hand strengthening sessions.

Focusing on this ball kept my mind from thinking about everything else that was taking place around me. It was a gift from my parents that not only served the purpose of reducing stress, but also kept my mind engaged with wanting to make progress. It was an object that symbolized a way to heal, and it was significant that it resembled the Earth, because this foam ball was slowly helping me get back to the world that I once knew.

Light

My room was very well lit at all times—from the sunshine coming through the window behind my bed to the fluorescent lights on the ceiling.

Over time I unknowingly built up my pain tolerance to the point where I was not even aware of being given a needle or a new IV. However, the pain tolerance did not impair my sense of hot or cold. I enjoyed the natural sunlight because I could feel its warmth on my pale and numb skin.

The sun was also a type of tracking device because I could decipher the day from the night by observing the sun's rays flickering against the walls. When the sun went down, the room was still incredibly bright from all the artificial lightbulbs, which added to the sensory overload that I was already experiencing. Even when I shut my eyes, the light still had a maddening way of penetrating the thin layer of my eyelids.

My sleeping pattern was drastically altered from the heavy medications, going in and out of consciousness, the constant beeping, being checked on and approached with needles or medication, and the omnipresent light. I understood that I had no control over any of these factors and that I was a sick patient who needed constant supervision. I appreciated the diligence of my care team. Their presence helped stimulate my mind and temporarily released it from my lonely existence. However, it would have greatly helped me to have the lights turned down at nighttime. I am not asking to completely turn the lights off, because that could be very dangerous, but to just lower the intensity. This measure would have had a profound impact on my sanity and also reduced my sleep deprivation. Turning the lights to a lower level would improve the patient's ability to achieve a night of high-quality rest.

Suggestions for Health Care Providers and/or Patient's Family:

- If there is a TV available in the room, keep it tuned to a station that you think the patient would like. Even if the volume is turned down, just having something visual patients can look at helps increase mental stimulation.

- Music soothes the soul. Even in dire situations, like a coma, hospitals could allow families to provide a patient's favorite music, within reason, as background noise, as long as it does not interfere with the medical equipment or the nurses' and doctors' work.

- If in doubt about the type of music to play for your loved one, classical music has been proven to bring about the most benefits for the patient, especially if he or she has anxiety, depressive syndromes, or are in pain or stressed (Trappe, 2010).

- If the care providers give permission, and if space is available in the patient's room, friends and family can post their letters and get well cards in an appropriate area.

- Family and friends can bring in photos they think the patient would like to see. It is a great way of bringing the patient's background into his or her new realm, because it can provide a sense of reassurance and hope that he or she can get life back to the way it was.

- When you bring in gifts for the patient, focus on bringing a token of encouragement that can be left in his or her room and seen by the patient and his or her visitors. Smaller items work well because they will not take up too much room; think quality, not quantity.

- Turn the lights down to a lower intensity throughout the night to help improve the sleep pattern of the patient.

Reflective Questions for Health Care Providers (write your answers in Part Five):

1) When you are taking care of the patient, how often are you reflecting on what he or she can possibly see, hear, and feel? What are some ways that you can help improve on this?

2) If there are TVs or radios available in the patient's room, do you prefer to keep them turned on or off? Can you describe a specific time when you saw a patient respond to his or her surroundings in a positive way when the TV or radio was turned on?

3) If you are working with patients who are long term or unable to drink fluids for a medical reason, how often do you proceed with measures related to mouth care?

4) If family and friends have brought in photos, get well cards, and other motivational items for the patient, do you ever find yourself looking at these items to get to know your patient better? Or, do you feel that viewing these items creates too much of a personal connection with the patient?

5) What are some specific ways that you help improve the patient's atmosphere to make it personal and relaxing for him or her?

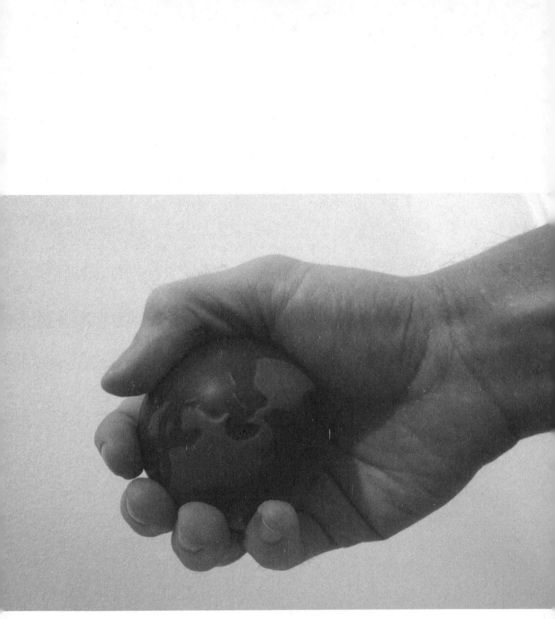

Squeezing the stress-relief ball was a useful way to regain strength and keep my mind off everything taking place around me.

CHAPTER 6

SETTING GOALS FOR THE PATIENT

IF YOU HAVE EVER TAKEN THE OPPORTUNITY TO WATCH THE OLYMPIC Games on television, you will have seen athletes from all over the world who want to represent their countries and be victorious over their competitors. You realize that these people who are appearing in front of you are 100 percent dedicated to what they do. Not only are they dedicated, but they are also determined. Determined to win, to succeed, and to prove to themselves that they can go beyond their limits and excel. They did not get to this point overnight; they spent most of their lives training and preparing, which is very similar to the way care providers train to do their best. You are personally inspired to go into the health care field; you go to school to get a proper education; you focus on a specialty that you would like to pursue and earn the necessary credentials; and you make the appropriate sacrifices until you achieve your goal of becoming a health care professional.

I am not a health care provider, or even an Olympic athlete, but I have learned many lessons about how important determination is while competing in sports for most of my life, especially during my endurance sports career, where I have participated in several marathons and Ironman triathlons. Over time, I realized that there are a lot of parallels with the way that I went through my physical therapy sessions and how I prepared for my endurance events, especially when it came to setting goals.

It is important to visualize what you would like your main goal to be and then write it down. After you have established this goal, the challenge is made and the pursuit begins. Do not put all your energy into thinking about how you are going to accomplish this goal, because it can be overwhelming in the very early stages, and you will get frustrated if you feel that you are making minimal progress along your path.

To help create a strong foundation in the beginning, it is effective to create smaller and achievable goals along the way—to track progress and boost confidence.

- After I started to slowly get back on my feet again, either my parents or my therapist would hold onto a restraint belt around my waist as I was relearning how to walk. Using a walker for support, I was able to make it about three or four feet before I felt the need to stop and sit down. My physical therapist and I plotted out the plan of how many feet we would like to accomplish over time. We had set our sights on the goal that I would be able to walk fifty feet at the end of five weeks of therapy, which was one of many goals.
- With this as the main goal, we broke down each week into ten-foot increments. The focus was not on walking fifty feet right away, but on walking ten feet farther than I had the previous week.

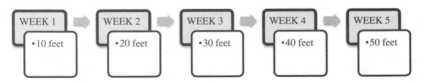

Weekly plan to increase walking distance.

Within each week, we put together a list of exercises and drills that would increase my strength and improve my balance, which would help me achieve the goal for that week. I was an ambitious patient, and I was in a hurry to see progress, so I would often do these exercises in my free time.

After the goal is accomplished for a specific week, you can set your sights on the following week and what measures you can take to make that happen. Everything is improving, the patient is getting stronger, you are continuously motivating the patient, confidence is building, and the patient is accomplishing the goals as planned.

Each week you continue to set your sights on improving just a little bit more. It is not the end of the world if your progress begins to plateau or slow down; setbacks can appear at any time. If this occurs, you should figure out how you can fix these problems and further motivate the patient in ways you think will benefit his or her outlook. Is this a medical concern? Is the patient getting enough rest between exercises and sessions? Is he or she eating a healthy diet? Are you putting forth the required effort to show improvements?

My support system of family and friends was a big inspiration when it came to setting goals. They gave me strength in times of weakness, and they kept me hopeful that tomorrow could be a better day. Unfortunately, not every patient is going to have a large support system that will provide encouragement when facing a challenge. As the care provider, you must do your best to represent his or her support system and motivate him or her to stay positive along the path to recovery.

You can frequently remind patients that both you and their entire care team believes in them. When they are feeling down, you can help lift their spirits up by commenting on something that they have recently accomplished during their recovery. When they feel that they will not be able to accomplish the goals they had set for themselves, try to have them focus on altering their approach to accomplishing those goals. Their path may not be the way they expected it to be, but you can help them understand that their life is not over and that this new path in life is just beginning. Through teamwork and perseverance, you will be able to help your patient achieve his or her short-term goals, which will ultimately lead to long-term goals.

When it comes to setting goals, the two most important things that I have learned is that anything is possible, and that any day is a great day when you live your dreams.

Suggestions for Health Care Providers and/or Patient's Family:

- Set realistic goals for the patient.
- Review the medical transfer file and consult with a doctor for any concerns.
- Monitor your patient closely—especially heart rate, respiratory rate, breathing pattern, temperature, and blood pressure.
- Do not put the patient in a situation where the patient could get injured.
- Reflect on your progress and improvements each week.
- Alter your plans accordingly if you see that the patient is well ahead or well behind the planned schedule.

Reflective Questions for Health Care Providers (write your answers in Part Five):

1) When you select a long-term goal for the patient, what are the steps you take in order to help the patient achieve it? (E.g., do

you break the long-term goal into smaller goals, do you focus only on the main goal, or do you have a long-term goal in mind but keep it only to yourself without letting the patient know about it?)

2) Think back on a specific time when a patient of yours was getting discouraged. What did you do or say to him or her to help cheer him or her up?

3) If you were the patient, what types of things would inspire you to accomplish your goals?

4) If you were the patient, what types of things would make you feel overwhelmed or pessimistic about achieving the stated goals?

5) If your patient is struggling to achieve goals, what is one way that you can encourage him or her to stay positive?

PART THREE

COMMUNICATION

"Watch your thoughts; they become words. Watch your
words; they become actions. Watch your actions; they
become habit. Watch your habits; they become character.
Watch your character; it becomes your destiny."

—Lao Tzu

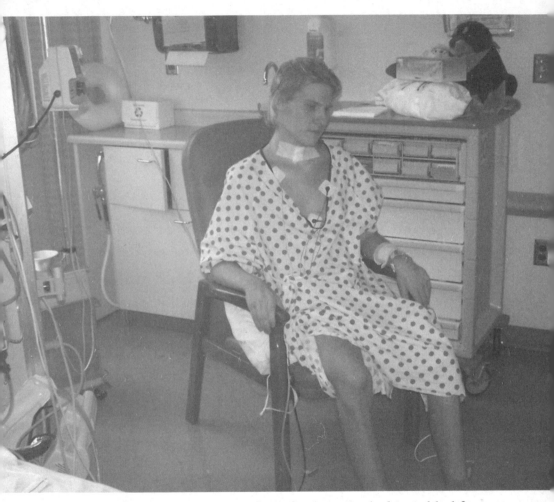

Slowly getting used to sitting in a chair after being in the hospital bed for two months. Each day we would increase the number of minutes to build up the endurance and stamina of my weakened muscles.

CHAPTER 7

BEFORE STEPPING INTO
THE PATIENT'S ROOM

As a medically induced comatose patient, I was coherent and very aware of my surroundings for a majority of my stay in the ICU. Whoever came into my room, I was instantly attuned to their presence, mood, actions, and, especially, their voice. It became a way of processing the information around me so I could better understand my situation.

My lack of mobility and limited line of sight were obstacles to consistently being able to see the people in my room. Even though my eyes may not have been directed toward them, I could still "see" them through momentary glimpses. Their moving shadows also helped me track them spatially throughout the room. It was the sound of their voices, shuffling papers, and their routine adjustments to my medical equipment that pinpointed their exact locations.

As time went on, I felt like my body was activating this hidden defense mechanism that I never knew I had—supersensory perception that I did not even know existed or was humanly possible. Every day this new skill was further developed and advanced, and in a way, became an important part of my survival.

I could even sense the positive or negative energy of the people who came into my room by their tone of voice, body language, gestures, and movement. I could immediately tell if they were having a good day or a really bad day, which was reflected in the treatment I received. I spent so much time with my team that I gradually learned their traits, common phrases, and mannerisms.

I have always been fascinated with the field of psychology since I took an introductory course my junior year in high school. My main interest involved what motivates our inner thoughts and actions. How do we perceive the external world, interpret it, and then follow up with a response? What triggers the decisions that we make?

In my place in the ICU, I was in a prime position to find the answers to some of these questions that I always pondered. I became a dedicated student of human nature in a real-world setting.

Even though I was the patient and constantly being supervised, I was also studying the behavior of my care providers and making my own observations about them. The way they carried themselves had a lot to do with their backgrounds and experiences, but especially with how they handled any unplanned stress that arose during the day.

I always hoped my providers were having a good day, because it created a positive atmosphere for me and the other staff working with them during that shift. Their cheerful presence was similar to the sun's power to create an illuminating ray of comfort on a cold and dreary day. With the first glimpse of that sunlight you are embraced with warmth. The same goes for being around people with positive attitudes. Just being near this type of person makes you feel better, and being with a negative person makes you feel sad.

A clear way to define this even further is to visualize an invisible barrier that separates the patient's room. Once you step into the room, the

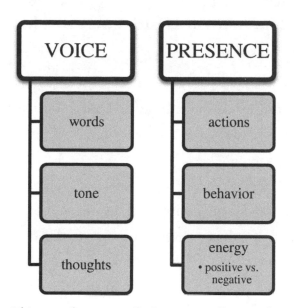

Things to be aware of when you walk into the patient's room.

full focus is directly on the health of the patient, along with your voice and presence within the room.

When you step out of the room, the focus is on everything else. Not only will this help the patient in the long run, but it will also allow for a reduction in distractions and potential medical errors.

Suggestions for Health Care Providers and/or Patient's Family:

- Every time you leave one room and enter another room, it is important to reground your thoughts.
- Focus on the greater good of caring for your patient.
- When you are having a chaotic day, think about a happy memory, sing a favorite song in your head, or do something that you know will distract your mind.

Reflective Questions for Health Care Providers (write your answers in Part Five):

1) When you are having a hectic day, what are some of the strategies that have helped you redirect your focus and energy?

2) What can you do to prepare yourself before walking into a patient's room?

3) After being given your report/sign-out on a patient with a family that has a reputation for being difficult, how can you prepare yourself to walk into that room with an unbiased opinion?

4) If you are having a bad day in your personal life, what can you do to compartmentalize your feelings in order to give completely dedicated care to your patient?

5) If you notice a coworker is having a stressful day through his or her words or actions, what can you do to help him or her make the appropriate change in his or her attitude and behavior?

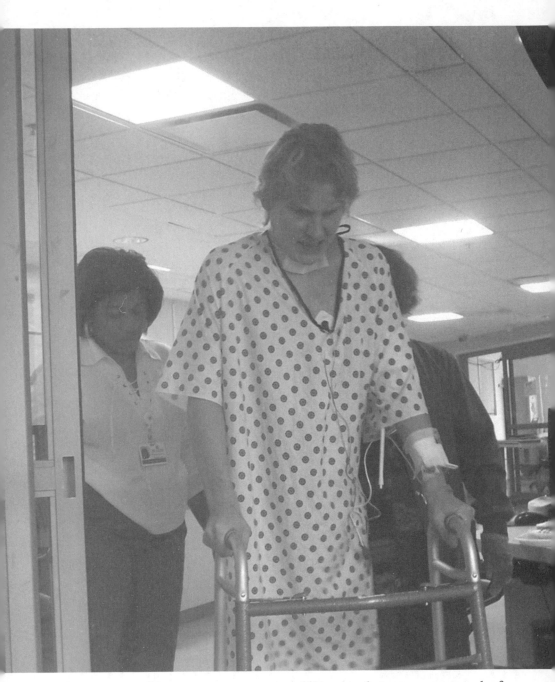

Taking my very first steps as my care team and parents cheer me on every inch of the way.

CHAPTER 8

BEDSIDE MANNERS ARE AS SIMPLE AS A SMILE

Throughout my recovery, whenever I was feeling down or depressed about my situation, my grandfather would offer me some encouraging words and remind me of the old saying that it takes more muscles to frown than to smile. I always wondered if this was scientifically proven, but any time he would remind me of this statement, I would always respond with a smile.

Smiling is important for a lot of reasons. It shows the people around you that you are happy, in a positive mood, and thankful that the day is going as you planned. Maybe you received good news, or it is one day closer to the weekend. Whatever the reason, I believe that when you smile, you just feel better and people like to be around people who are in a good mood. I do not know if it is a sensitivity that we have based on our muscle memory and subconscious responses, but I definitely prefer this simple expression compared to the alternative of frowning.

The first thing I noticed when a new nurse, doctor, therapist, or medical assistant walked into my room was whether he or she smiled within the first few minutes of being around me. My spirits soared when I saw a cheerful facial expression on his or her face, and I was concerned if I saw a frown or nothing at all.

Throughout the week, my doctors would make their rounds within the unit and discuss the patient's progress with his or her family or review treatment with the medical teams on that shift.

On one occasion I can remember watching the ICU director walking around with his medical students from a local university. I always looked forward to seeing him, especially when I relearned how to talk again, because I was starving for conversation and his presence always brightened my day.

When he and his group of a dozen medical students stopped in front of my room, he had a big smile on his face. The medical students stared at me with nervous expressions behind their clipboards. He greeted me with a thumbs-up and asked how I was doing, explained that he had just talked to my parents outside the unit, and how he was thrilled with the progress I was making. Our conversation was upbeat as always and his words were incredibly motivational to me.

The entire group walked a few steps farther into my room and the director gave the medical students a detailed rundown of my background, injuries, health updates, and progress. As he spoke to them using medical terminology I could not decipher, I smiled at the students and waved to them, feeling a bit vulnerable. They stood there, looking at me, frozen in time, and listening to him. They wrote down notes on their clipboards and glanced at the medical equipment in my room without ever acknowledging me. Then I just felt like I should cover my face with the bedsheet or go hide in a closet somewhere.

I know that an ICU is a serious environment full of critically ill patients, and students are under a lot of pressure from their schoolwork.

I gave them the benefit of the doubt and tried to engage them in friendly conversation to put them at ease during their visit with me. They were only a few years older than me so I wanted to meet them on their level. I ventured a "hello."

A deafening silence filled the air, and blood rushed to my face in embarrassment. They continued staring at me, looking around at each other to see if anyone would find the courage to respond. They glanced over at the director, and he encouraged them to say hello to me. I then asked how they were doing. Again, there was nothing, except for a young guy who nodded at me. That was it, an awkward nod. My attempt at conversation with the students was over, and I was embarrassed to have initiated this interaction in the first place.

I existed in this state only as a body to be studied. From limb to limb, and head to toe, I was a collection of anatomical charts and medical diagrams to these young men and women. A textbook example, in living form. But I was so much more than that.

I like to think that maybe it was their first time doing rounds in the ICU with a doctor. Maybe they were so used to seeing other, unconscious patients in the unit that they were not quite expecting to see a patient sitting up, making eye contact, and trying to talk to them. Or perhaps they were just shy individuals who were so engaged in learning how to treat the body that they had not quite made it to the area in their studies where they learn how to heal the person. Whatever the reason, I hoped that they would learn a little bit more about the importance of bedside manners before they started treating patients in their medical careers.

When it comes to the recovery of the patient, why is it so important that the care provider have an effective bedside manner? There is so much going on in the hospital room; who has the time to worry about something like that when people's lives are hanging by a thread? It's because something as simple as a smile represents more than just a facial expression in the hospital. It is a symbol of compassion, of hope, of support.

For a patient, a smile can be a visual response as monumental as blinking or lifting a finger on command. It can help show signs of life in a patient when the only thing that may have appeared before was darkness. On the other end of the spectrum, a care provider who smiles is visually showing people that he or she is nice, caring, approachable, and compassionate.

This does not mean that caregivers who wear blank expressions are unfriendly, but positive first impressions do matter to the patient and family. The patient wants to feel secure and know that he or she is in good hands with the care team. The family wants their care provider to be someone who is friendly and easy to interact with without ever feeling intimidated. In the deepest and darkest moments of human suffering, a simple smile can go a very long way.

BEDSIDE MANNERS

- Address patient by name
- Shake patient's hand when appropriate
- Maintain eye contact
- Assume a relaxed posture
- Do not appear to be in a rush
- Listen to the patient and the family
- Address any concerns
- Smile

Suggested bedside manners for care providers.

Suggestions for Health Care Providers and/or Patient's Family:

- Think about the impact you are making in the lives of your patients and their families.
- Be positive and optimistic around your patients and their families.
- Do not be afraid to talk to your patients.
- Always be aware of the importance of bedside manners when you engage with a patient and his or her family.

Reflective Questions for Health Care Providers (write your answers in Part Five):

1) How would you rate your bedside manners?
2) What is one recommendation that you can give to brand-new care providers on how to initiate a conversation with a patient?
3) How can you personally convey to the patient that he or she is not just a body being treated, but a person?
4) When you walk into the room of a new patient, is there a certain protocol (e.g., smile, shake hands, address by first name, sit down next to him or her) that you follow in order to make the patient feel comfortable in your presence?
5) If you were the patient, what is something that your care provider could do to make you feel at ease?

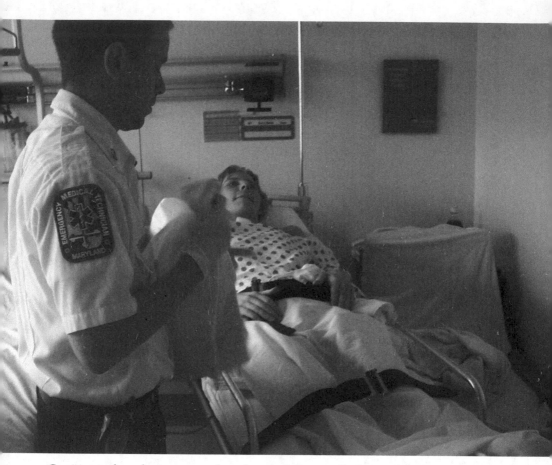

Getting ready to be transported to the rehabilitation facility. I always appreciated when my care providers would take the time to explain what they were doing when it came to my treatment plan.

CHAPTER 9

TALKING TO THE PATIENT AND HIS OR HER FAMILY

It can be lonely in the hospital for a patient and his or her family, especially in the ICU. Any form of conversation or mental stimulation is very meaningful, because it provides a temporary relief for the patient and comfort for the family. Talking to the patient, whatever his or her background or situation, is critical because it creates a solid foundation of trust—whether the patient is conscious or unconscious, in a good mood or bad mood, or cooperative or not. The health care provider is in a prime position to make a positive impact and provide ongoing motivational support.

Glanz, Rimer, and Viswanath discuss the ways that communication between the care provider and patient can affect health outcomes in their book, *Health Behavior and Health Education: Theory, Research, and Practice*. "Clinician-patient communication can affect health directly or can affect it indirectly through the mediating effects of proximal outcomes such as greater mutual understanding, trust, patient satisfaction, and patient involvement in decision making."

The health care providers who stood out to us were the individuals who not only did an amazing job in taking care of my medical needs, but went a step further by focusing on the emotional and psychological well-being of me and my parents. These hardworking men and women walked into my room with a smile on their faces on a daily basis, addressed me by my name, read my get well cards on the wall, and spoke to my family. There was a sense of trust developing each time we saw them. In my eyes they had quickly become the health care system's version of the "dream team." I looked forward to seeing my dream team members. They were always in a good mood, and that was contagious. Even at times when my visual field was restricted to the ceiling or a wall in my room, I could instantly recognize their uplifting energy. They had become my friends, even though I was not able to speak to them. They had a lot going on, but they took the time to talk to us.

In his book, *Better: A Surgeon's Notes on Performance*, Dr. Atul Gawande discusses how it is very important to initiate conversations, especially in the hospital, because care providers can learn about the people they are working with every day, both coworkers and patients. "You don't have to come up with a deep or important question, just one that lets you make a human connection." A simple interaction can make the atmosphere that much more pleasant.

There were many days in the hospital when my health was slipping and my parents desperately needed a helping hand or a shoulder to cry on. My care providers were not just taking care of me, they were also taking care of my family. The communication from the doctors and nurses really kept my parents going.

Our nurses and doctors would talk about my condition and surgeries that were needed or answer any questions my parents had when they were available. The nurses were a wealth of information because they were with me for long periods of time, and they would forewarn my family of potential issues we would face each day. One gave us the scenario that "if Brian makes it through the first hours, twenty-four and then forty-eight, the next phase will be a roller-coaster ride, and the ups and downs will be rough." During the patient's hospitalization, nurses are in a key position to support family members, maintain family integrity, and ready them for assuming the role of caretaker during the patient's recovery (Van Horn & Kautz, 2007). We were a family that had never been in this type of situation before, and having someone there to help explain things and offer support made a world of difference.

During my stay in the ICU, visiting hours were in three one-hour intervals, in the morning (11 a.m.), early afternoon (2 p.m.), and again at night (7 p.m.). My parents were there, on average, ten hours a day, not including an hour drive to and from home every day. They both worked and had to take leaves of absence, which also hurt us financially. They found places around the hospital to sit, especially the outside spaces. They later told me that the one question they would never ask each other was, "Do you think Brian is going to die?" They constantly thought it, but could never bring themselves to say it out loud.

My parents felt bad the first couple of days after the accident, because family and friends were coming to the hospital to say what we thought were last "good-byes." The nurses told them that even though I was in a comatose state, having people in the room would overstimulate me, and they had to administer more and more medication. In fact, some of the nurses would ask a visitor to leave if they stirred things up in my room. It was hard because everyone was hurting, and people react differently to sad and desperate situations. My parents found it difficult having to face the same questions over and over again, especially when neither they nor my medical team had any answers.

My parents were my first visitors every morning, and they could tell early on how the day would go based on which nurse I had (all my care providers were good, but some were great because they went above and beyond with their nursing care). After confronting a dispiriting scene in my room, coming out to the waiting room to face everyone was excruciating. They were bombarded with questions about my status and who would get to go in next, and then visitors complained that people were taking too long. My parents had life-and-death decisions to make, and the last thing they wanted to deal with was upsetting visitors. Some would even interfere with the doctors and nurses doing their jobs. Then it all seemed to become a social event. They finally had to ask everyone to leave after I made it through the first week. It was a very difficult thing for my parents to do, and it meant a lot to them to have so much support, but they wanted to focus 100 percent on me and my situation. They could not worry about who was upset or what everyone was saying.

Day after day, my parents saw patients come and go while I remained. They talked with other family members going through the same sadness and ambiguous situations. But as days went on, my parents retreated into a type of solitude. They had each other, and the focus was on me. Families are all different. These are the types of situations that can make or break people and families.

According to a study by Livesay, Mokracek, Sebastian, and Walsh (2005), a group of twenty-six registered nurses (RN) and patient care assistants (PCA) were interviewed regarding their perceptions of the impact of visiting hours on the progress of the patient. They reported that some of the benefits of visiting hours included decreased blood pressure, heart rate, and intracranial pressure (ICP). In certain situations, visiting hours can show negative results, such as increased anxiety, a change in vital signs, or a decrease in mental activity. The staff believed that the benefits of the visiting hours were specific to the family and patient and dependent on the hospital's visitation policy.

Telephone calls were another major form of communication. Night-time was difficult both because my parents were unable to meet the night nurses to form a comfortable bond with them and because some calls were frightening since my health was fading in and out constantly. A nurse would call early in the morning and late at night to give my parents an updated status report; the phone call at night was helpful, but they said it would have been nice to meet some of the night nurses to say "thank you." It was agony waiting for the calls. Most of the time, the information was not good, but they would take what they could get. I was still alive, and that was the main thing. That phone call was a valuable tool to keep them informed, since they would leave at night not knowing if there would be a tomorrow. Once they got home, they would silently wait for the phone calls.

After two months and two days, I was transferred to a rehabilitation facility. It was evident from the moment we moved in that this phase was not going to be like our excellent hospital stay. Communication was lacking from the day I moved in. Mom and Dad chose this place after an earlier meeting set up by a social worker from my hospital. The facility was nice, the staff was informative, and the outdoor space was beautiful. Being outside was the key for us. Fresh air, open space, and sunshine were a far cry from the ICU.

Although we were elated to be leaving the hospital, we were also very nervous. I was leaving a safe place to go to an unknown one. Could my health withstand leaving my safe zone? It felt like I was leaving home for the first time, because my medical team had become my family. After we said our good-byes with huge hugs and tears, I was cautiously loaded into the ambulance. Mom and Dad followed behind for the drive to the center. They had reserved a room at the local hotel, because they were not allowed to stay at the facility with me. Initially, that was a deterrent for them, but now they would not face that long commute, as they preferred to stay near me. Our insurance allowed a five-day stay at the rehab facility, but considering what I had been through and my body's condition, we thought this should have been longer.

When we arrived in the early evening, there was no one to greet us or show us the way. Even the front desk did not seem to know we were coming. After some time, they moved us to a room in the spinal injury section very far from anyone on staff or any other patients. The ambulance guys carefully moved me from the stretcher to one of the beds in the room. The other bed was empty. My parents prepared to leave as visiting hours were coming to a close, and then I began vomiting. There was no one around to help me, and at that moment my parents refused to leave me alone. The nurse came in to say our time was over and that they could not stay. They refused and slept across the room in the empty bed. They were afraid that if I continued vomiting, I would choke, or worse. It was only days that I had been out of my coma, and my body was not well.

The next few days included physical therapy, occupational therapy, and speech/cognitive therapy. It was hard, but I worked to the best of my ability. The physical therapy sessions were not easy, because I was so weak and my blood pressure would skyrocket. As a result, the therapist thought I was stressed. Since my parents refused to leave me alone, one was allowed to stay overnight. The rehab center wanted to move me to another room with seven guys until another room opened up, but my parents became upset and the facility moved me to a single room. So, in a five-day stay, I was moved to three different rooms. My parents did not want to cause any problems but they wanted to be there at all times, even if just one could stay.

After five days, it was time to go home. A doctor came in to prepare the discharge papers and noticed I should have been on blood pressure medication. According to the physical therapist, I was stressed when I could not get through my sessions and had to sit because of my heart rate being elevated. How come the therapist did not review my records or talk to a doctor about my situation? What did this person know about my condition? My parents and I would have been comforted to have better communication.

I really was not in any condition to go home, but after all we had been through as a family, we were ready—if a little scared. The experience going from a hospital with amazing quality of care, compassion for me, the patient, as well as my family and friends, and extensive communication from all levels, left my parents and me feeling empty in the rehabilitation environment. We are not people who are negative, but we also cannot sugarcoat things that could have been better.

Once we were home, the outpatient rehabilitation facility we chose was excellent and communication was spot on. The different therapists briefed us on the initial phase of their plan and kept us informed each week. They cared about us. So for the next four months, three times a week, we all worked together as a team toward my progress. Times were tough, but each step forward would bring better results. There were setbacks, so we took each day as a positive and went from there.

The power that care providers have extends beyond medically treating the patient. This power is based on building a solid bond between themselves and the patient where further progress can take place. In the innovational book, *Critical Decisions: How You and Your Doctor Can Make the Right Medical Decisions Together*, Dr. Peter Ubel states, "To properly collaborate with patients in making difficult medical decisions, doctors need to not only communicate complicated information in ways that patients will comprehend but also anticipate the way patients are likely to respond to their words." Most of my care providers explained exactly what they were doing when they were doing it, but they went beyond just stating the facts, because they knew how my parents and I would react. In order to provide the best type of care, the care providers took the time to get to know me, my family, my past, and my present. While doing so, they were shaping my future.

I highly encourage you to talk to your patients as often as you can, whether they can hear you or not. I know I could hear my surroundings, and I was grateful for any interaction at all. Even if the patient is comatose or physically unresponsive, there is always that chance that he or she can hear you. It may be only a brief amount of time, or even just a few seconds, but key changes could be taking place during those few seconds. It is extremely important to make the attempt as often as possible, because these conversations can bring forth drastic improvements in the patient's recovery and trigger the mental stimulation that can encourage a response and potential improvement.

So what are recommended topics to talk about with your patients and their families?

Break the Ice

It depends on the person and his or her background, but the biggest step is to just break the ice and start a conversation. Talking to the patient about something casual like the weather is always a good start, because the patient can think of the outside world and momentarily break free from a confined realm of existence. You can provide the patient with small details about what it is like outside or about the forecast. The more visual imagery, the better; the patient can allow the imagination to run wild.

But what if the patient is unresponsive or comatose? You can still talk to the patient, and you should as often as you can. He or she may not be able to show comprehension visually, but you have to at least make the attempt. Even if you have a conversation with yourself—talk about your background, interests, things you have in common, weekend plans—it will still be a great benefit for the patient. Not only will your words stimulate the patient's mind, but you are also strengthening the bond of trust that you have with him or her, which will be of great importance in the long run.

But what if there is little to no brain activity? In my personal experience, and from hearing the experiences of others, I still feel that it is very important to talk to these patients.

My grandmother was diabetic with an extensive medical history and underwent a quadruple bypass surgery in the mid-1990s. Even after the surgery, her health was still a concern to the family, and visits to the hospital became routine. On a hot summer day in 2006, she went into cardiac arrest as she walked into her cardiologist's office for a routine appointment. They were able to revive her after several minutes, but for the next several days she was in a coma with extremely limited brain activity. Her coma was not medically induced like mine, and she was not showing any reliable responses to the tests that they were running, which was a big concern to her health care team and our family.

Even though the results of her medical scans were not positive, I reflected on my time as a patient and thought about the things that helped improve my experience. I made sure that we brought in a small stereo to play her favorite music, I opened the blinds in her windows to let in the sunshine, I read get well cards to her out loud, I turned the television to programs that I knew she enjoyed, and most importantly, I talked to her every chance I had. I did not want to monopolize the situation and take away visiting time from the rest of the family, but I just made sure that her environment was as comfortable as possible and encouraged everyone to talk to her as much as they could about happier times. It was very difficult to be positive in a heartbreaking situation like this, but everyone did his or her best to be upbeat and put on a happy face.

After she had already been in the hospital for a few days, I thought it would be appropriate to read my grandmother a letter I had written for her birthday to see if I could get any reaction at all. I stood next to my grandmother's bed, holding her hand. My grandmother's eyes directly faced mine, and as I stared into her bright blue eyes, I desperately tried to find any signs of life that remained.

I started reading the letter to her, and the pure intensity of the moment brought tears to my eyes. As I continued, something amazing happened: tears also started streaming down her face, her eyes gently blinked, and she moved her mouth as if she were trying to say something to console me, as if trying to tell me that I did not need to be sad and that everything was going to be okay.

Up until that moment, she had not shown any signs similar to this, and any responses that she made to commands were extremely faint and not purposeful. After that afternoon, unfortunately, her health continued to fail and we had to take her off life support later that week. During this difficult ordeal, the memory of her response to my letter brought me peace and closure. As I read to her, I knew that she was there with me and was acknowledging my presence, even for just a few seconds.

You should never assume that the patient is unable to hear because the mind and body are extraordinarily resilient. From my personal experience, and from the dozens of stories I have heard from other patients and care providers over the years, there is always a chance that the patient is aware of what is taking place around him or her.

Get Well Cards

Reading aloud the patient's get well cards can also have such an influence on his or her outlook. Due to the personal nature of the cards, it is a good idea to get permission from the family so you can find the cards you feel are suitable and will have the greatest impact.

Patients need all the motivation they can get, especially from the people they are closest to, and reading their cards is a beneficial tactic to keep them from becoming depressed. If someone sent a card in the first place, there is a pretty good chance that a solid friendship or bond exists between them. The stronger that bond, the more of an impact the letter can make when the patient is feeling down.

Treatment Information

I listened when my medical team would take the time to explain what they were doing in my medical treatment. I was not interested in all the advanced details or specific medical terminology, but I liked hearing a comprehensible explanation of their actions. Whether it was drawing blood, traveling to the radiology department, taking an X-ray, or giving me a new IV or type of medication, I wanted to be updated on anything and everything that was happening around me. I needed just enough information to know what was taking place and that they were taking care of me.

My care providers would regularly discuss my health updates so they would all be on the same page if they had to work with me during the week. On occasion, I would overhear the serious details of my own prognosis—often frightening news, as I was one of the sickest patients in the ICU for most of my time there. On the roller-coaster ride of ups and downs, I was usually on the dreaded uphill climb with no end in sight. I knew my health was questionable, but I did not want to overhear detailed conversations about it right in front of me. This was both a frustrating and terrifying occurrence. As a patient who might be able to obtain only external information by listening, even a conversation that is taking place right outside the hospital room has the potential of being heard.

I believe any conversation that takes place within the patient's room, in any department of the hospital, should be focused away from the patient's prognosis. Talking to patients, rather than about them (and their health statuses), is important. The conversation should stay within the realms of helping to improve the patient's overall quality of living, orienting the patient to his or her location, explaining the measures being taken to care for the patient, and giving an occasional motivational boost. The more conversation, the more it will stimulate patients' minds. If the patient is unresponsive there is still a chance of breaking through to him or her.

I also appreciated getting to know my care providers as individuals rather than just as the dedicated people taking care of me each day. I overheard conversations about my health care team's personal lives and plans for the weekend, which I enjoyed because I could momentarily reflect back on my life doing similar fun activities. I was also able to gain a better understanding of their personalities, like whether they were generally optimistic or pessimistic.

There is no exact science or perfect method of talking to your patients, but you should try to make a connection through communication. Once that link is made, you can potentially guide them out of that darkness.

Daily Topics in the News

A good way to engage the patient as a person and keep him or her in the loop is to mention topics in the daily news. In most circumstances, life tends to go on standby for the patient and family until the patient's condition improves. Even if some progress is made, it can be a very slow process to reenter the world. From my experiences, a feeling of being left behind can develop and one's personality may never be the same after that.

In May of 2004, I had just graduated with honors from high school and I was preparing for my freshman year in college. The morning of the accident, I was at swim practice training for my first year on the college team. As a family, our world stopped around 1:15 p.m. on July 6 and did not start spinning again until I began showing signs of progress in the hospital. Even then, it took years for us to get back into the regular rhythm of life again. From our own experience, along with the dozens of conversations that I have had with families that have experienced such tragedy and adversity in their lives, we share a similar perspective on the world. Updating a patient on the goings-on of the day could help him or her feel connected with the living world.

Optimistic Word Choice

Using optimistic words or phrases is critical when patients are often scared and worried. Positive reinforcement not only is helpful, but helps build a safe haven in an unknown place and allows for a steady progression to take place.

For instance, in the moments when I was so weak that I could not even twitch a finger or blink on command, some of my nurses would encourage me several times a day to follow their simple commands. They would gently wean me off the heavy sedation, hold my hand, and in an uplifted voice say, "Can you blink for me today, Brian? I know you can, I know you have it in you. Squeeze my hand just a little bit. You can do it!"

It was a very motivational effort on their part, and they would not give up on me. They wanted to see me succeed, and some of my care providers would even add some humor into the mix. "Come on, Brian, everyone here is working so hard to get you better. I'll leave you alone if you blink for me or squeeze my hand. As soon as you do it, I'll stop bugging you."

In that moment, I looked at their determined smiles and reflected on their motivational support. They believed in me, and I did not want to let them down. I wanted to escape my locked-in state as rapidly as I could, so I used all my strength to follow their simple commands. I do not know where the inner strength came from, but after many routines like this, I was finally able to fulfill their simple requests.

Life Experiences

When talking to patients, you should think of something that you believe might interest them. If you know a little bit about their lives and experiences from talking to their families and friends, this helps engage their interest. Whether they like sports, riding horses, traveling, quilting, or staying at home and watching their favorite movies, you are tapping into something that intrigues them and establishing that necessary line of communication. You are reaching out to them and entering their world, but you are also showing compassion for their individuality, which strengthens that communication and the feeling of trust.

Suggestions for Health Care Providers and/or Patient's Family:

- Extending ICU visiting hours could be a target for review, depending on the condition of the patient.
- Allow a family to meet the night nurse during a specified time.
- It would be helpful if there were a hospital computer system where a family representative could check medical information and the status of a patient.
- Have someone to guide patients when arriving at a rehab facility. Have the person, or the team of people, working with a patient discuss his or her medical condition, prescriptions, and rehabilitation plan so they are all on the same page when communicating with family members.
- Similar to patient and family engagement in the hospital setting, the family members could add valuable pieces of information regarding the patient in rehab.
- When you are in the patient's room, whether you know it or not, you are already interacting with him or her. A single word does not have to be spoken for an interaction to occur, but audible conversation does have a profound impact on the thoughts and feelings of the patient.
- Helping a family feel accepted by the hospital staff can be initiated by making eye contact, talking with the family, and listening to their questions (Browning & Warren, 2006).

- Have a printout or computer log the patient's family can reference, even in emergency or ICU situations, to help them understand what is going on. Some people may find it helpful to view the medical records during their hospital stay, and it may help the healing process along.

Reflective Questions for Health Care Providers (write your answers in Part Five):

1) When you first started working as a care provider, how did you feel the first time you interacted with the patient and his or her family? How do you feel now when you talk to them? If there has been a change over the years, why do you think this is?

2) When you witness a visitor interact with the patient, what are the signs that the patient enjoys or dislikes the presence of the visitor?

3) What are your favorite topics that you enjoy discussing with your patients and their families?

4) Is there any particular method of communication that you feel works well with patients and their families? What methods tend not to work?

5) What is one particular thing that you can start doing right away to improve your communication with your patients and their families?

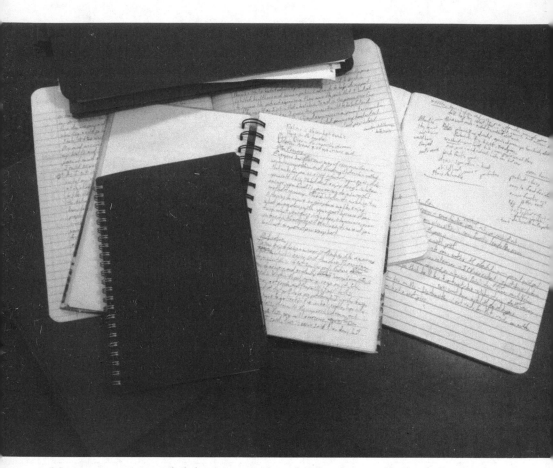

My nurses recommended that I put my thoughts down in a journal to help with the psychological recovery. These are a few of the composition books that I would pour my heart and soul into every day.

CHAPTER 10

KEEPING A JOURNAL

COMMUNICATION IN THE HOSPITAL ROOM IS MUCH MORE THAN SPOKEN words or body language; it can also be the written word. Keeping a journal is a great way to track progress during the recovery process, both for the patient and family members.

It was a challenge to go from twenty-four-hour observational care in the ICU to a rehab center where you are checked on only occasionally. I was bedridden, dependent, and extremely weak, so I needed my parents to stay with me at all times. I was learning how to transition from my hospital bed to a wheelchair, and my parents were learning how to become my full-time nurses.

I participated in several physical and occupational therapy sessions during the days at the rehab center. I had a lot of downtime in between my outpatient therapy sessions, and I spent most of this time quietly reflecting on the previous months. I was still trying to piece together the entire situation, and I had a lot of questions for my parents about my two-month stay in the hospital, about the extent of my injuries, and about the day of the accident.

My parents had a very difficult time talking about these topics, and they started to show visible signs of post-traumatic stress disorder

(PTSD) as soon as we arrived at the rehab center. This was understandable, and I knew how much they had been through. They had spent the last two months trying to be hopeful in a hopeless situation. Living each day, not knowing if I would live or die, took its toll.

They often say that you do not know how strong people are until you see them at their weakest moments, and the inner and outer strength that my parents displayed never faltered. They did their best to put on a brave face to all those around them, including me. Their strength gave me strength—especially in the moments when I thought about giving up.

When I was transferred to the rehab center, we were one step closer to going home, and the suppressed rush of emotions from the past two months started to come to the surface for my parents. Everything they had tried to conceal and forget was starting to return to their minds. Just by looking at their facial expressions I could instantly tell that they were reflecting on painful memories.

I did my best to keep the conversations focused on pleasant things—how it was so nice to be able to go outside for fresh air, how I could not wait to go home, and how I was excited to see my family and friends and show them the progress I was making. However, disguised behind my positive tone and conversations, I was trying my best to absorb a lot of information and emotions.

I had both good and bad days, and I tried to stay optimistic around my parents, even though some days it was not easy. I did not want to show any signs that I was having difficulty or feeling down about my current physical state, because I knew it would worry them. Even a cough or a sneeze would draw concerned looks. I tried to keep a smile on my face at all times, because I understood the cheerful impact it would have on them.

After I was released from the rehab center, it was a new type of transition as I became accustomed to living at home again. Due to my limited strength, I could not walk around the house without assistance nor could I go upstairs. My bed and some of my furniture from my room were brought downstairs to the living area, which became my temporary room for the first month at home.

It was a new experience to finally be back in the place where I grew up, surrounded by great childhood memories and interacting with all the things that reminded me of my life before the accident. I still had a long way to go in my recovery, but I was so happy to be home.

I had some minor setbacks within the first few weeks, and I was readmitted to the hospital in early November to get checked out and receive some antibiotics. I was hoping to return to the hospital as a visitor, rather than as a patient, but I was happy to return in a wheelchair this time.

During my short-term stay, I was able to see a lot of my ICU care providers who had watched over me during the summer. I was also able to match a face to some of the providers who took care of me whom I had never met, although I had heard their names on many occasions while I was considered unresponsive. Even though I was in the hospital for less than a week, it felt more like a reunion with the various members from my care team. I had dozens of heartwarming conversations with my nurses, therapists, doctors, and surgeons about the progress I had been making up until that point, and they were ecstatic to see that I was regaining back some of my weight and rebuilding my strength.

They asked me how I was recovering physically, and I responded that things were steadily progressing. When they asked me how I was doing emotionally and psychologically, I had to ponder for a moment before I could respond. I knew I had a lot of thoughts running through my mind, but I guess I never truly stopped and thought about this until then. I realized that I was constantly wondering about the meaning behind all these life-altering situations that my family and I went through. Psychologically, I was still healing in a lot of ways, and my road to recovery was more than just a physical adaptation to regaining independence in the real world.

My nurses gave me a suggestion that changed my life then and there—I should record my thoughts in a journal. They explained that if I put my emotions on paper, I could work through a lot of the trauma I had been dealing with.

I explained it was too hard to talk about what I was going through with my parents, which they understood. In my journal, I would be the only reader. The goal was to fill each page with my inner thoughts, feelings, emotions, fears, concerns, and doubts, and there were no taboo topics, because the goal was to reflect, confront, and react to the information at hand. I could also log my physical therapy so I could clearly track the progress from day to day, and week to week. If in week one I could walk only ten feet, and in week two I could walk eleven feet, the journal would serve as a record of these improvements and provide an ongoing sense of hope and motivation.

My parents thought keeping a journal was a great idea. They told me about the online journal my friends and family had logged into to see my daily health updates and explained how they typically had focused on positive updates. These journal entries had provided my parents with hope about my situation; if I created a journal, I could possibly give myself hope.

As soon as I made it back home, I started pouring my heart and soul into a black-and-white composition book every chance I had. The act of putting a worry down on paper made me feel better. Some things took a little bit longer to come to terms with, but I felt that writing was a conscious and even subconscious effort to control and relieve any anxiety that I had.

The journal became an aid for me to push through the days when I was having a difficult time adjusting to my new life. If I did not have this outlet, I am quite certain that I would have also dealt with PTSD like my parents. Laughter may be the best medicine, but writing in my journal was great therapy for what I was going through.

As my stack of journals grew to be a foot high, I felt that my experiences could help others going through a similar bout of adversity. Thinking of these people is what ultimately inspired me to pursue the path of getting my journals published into a memoir. Whether an individual, family member, or friend, it was my sincere hope that my experiences could make a positive impact on those who were doing their best to overcome their own traumas and tragedies. My journals were transformed into my published book, *Iron Heart*, in 2009. The letters, emails, and messages I have received from readers are everything I had hoped they would be.

Below is a sample of my very first journal entry that I wrote when I was released from the hospital—for the second time—in November 2004. The entry documents my initial thoughts and memories of what it was like to wake up in the ICU.

Journal Entry—November 20, 2004

I awake to the sound of screaming, crying, and the loss of all reality. I then come to realize that I am in a white room all by myself. I have only been asleep for a short while, I think. From what I remember, it has been the only time that I have slept in the past few days, or has it been weeks? Where am I? I blink my eyes a few times and wait for them to adjust to the blinding light shining all around me. My eyes remain fixated on the dizzying blur of my bizarre surroundings.

My heart is racing and I am sweating profusely. I am completely numb all over, but I feel an overwhelming sense of pain. I cannot pinpoint what area of my body hurts the most; the agony penetrates all the way to the bone. The pain increases. I am so uncomfortable. The pain feels like a thousand needles stabbing me over and over. I feel like sandpaper has scraped off my skin. I try to move my fingers, but they seem to be in some kind of mitten that completely covers my hands. My arms are tied down as well, but why? What is going on, and what am I doing here?

I really cannot see straight, nor can I sense anything other than a fan to my right, by the wall. Its slight breeze does not cool my skin. I am extremely hot, and I can just feel beads of sweat dripping from my forehead. Fire is spreading through my veins. I feel like I am spontaneously combusting, and I am waiting for my body to just burst into flames at any second. My throat is sore. Everything is a blur. I am motionless and alone. I feel as if I am at the dentist, getting a cavity fixed, and they have put me on a high dose of nitrous oxide. If I could scream I would. I would scream from down deep until my vocal cords would bleed.

The night before remains nothing but a mystery to me. I do not know how long I have been residing within this room. I am starting to become mentally and physically weak. Am I dying or am I dreaming this? The people who come in the room tell me that I was in a car accident, but that does not make any bit of sense to me. How could I have been in an accident? I do not remember this happening. It just does not make sense. As I think about it, I come to the conclusion that I must have been a passenger because surely I was not the one driving. I am a safe and cautious driver, how could something like this happen to me?

My eyes continue to wander as I try to piece together the situation that I am in. The walls within this twelve-by-twelve room are crowded with electrical monitors and medical instruments. This must be pretty serious. There is an opening in the doorway at the front of my bed that brings in this intense light from the large room in front of me.

There is a clock above the doorway, and a chair to the right of me. There is no form of entertainment, like cards or board games that I could possibly occupy myself with. In truth, it would not even matter, because I cannot move. I do see a small TV in the upper right corner of my room, but it is turned off. What use is that? It is as if I am a prisoner in some kind of dark dungeon, completely paralyzed, with no plan of escape. But why am I here?

As days go by, I notice that I must be in a hospital because several people come in each day in blue uniforms and white coats to give me a specific dosage of medicine. What are they trying to cure with this medication? People come in to check on me and see how I am doing every few minutes. My vision is blurry so I cannot see the details of their faces, but I sense their presence. My hearing is muffled from the beeping sounds, and the haze of existence that I seem to be living in. I cannot respond to their questions. I feel like a zombie, because I just stare at everyone who comes in and walks by. I sense that I have some kind of a tube going down my throat and it hurts to swallow. All I can think about is having something to drink.

I do not know which hospital I am at, and that kind of feeling is not a good one to have. Am I anywhere near where I grew up? Am I even in the country?

The days go by in an instant. The clothing that I wear was provided by the hospital—a loose blue-and-white gown. I am able to catch only a glimpse of it when I am being moved around my bed or transported to a stretcher. I feel like my hair has grown down to my shoulders, my skin feels very dry, and my teeth are very gritty. What I would do to just take a nice shower and brush my teeth. My ectomorphic body is withering away ever so slowly. I am fed with some sort of liquid that goes into the tube down my throat. There might even be a tube that goes down my nose, too, but most of my face is still numb. I would pull these aggravating tubes out, but my arms are constantly strapped down.

I have lost the will to do anything but lie here on my back. This is how I continue my existence in the world for the time being. I stare at the light that is in front of me, and try to figure out the situation that I am in at the moment. What have I done to get in here? I do not remember anything happening to me so what is the reason for me staying here? My mind is blank to what may have happened. Am I alive or dreaming this? Please, somebody wake me up, I am begging you.

Suggestions for Health Care Providers and/or Patient's Family:

- Encourage the patient to keep a journal to track physical, emotional, and psychological progress and write down things that he or she may have a difficult time talking about.

- You do not have to be a patient to keep a journal. It is very effective for a family member or friend of somebody who is going through the recovery process. It is also effective for a care provider to keep a journal in order to reflect on certain patients, your interactions with them, and the overall outcomes of the people that you treat.

- The style of the journal is completely up to the writer. Do not worry about punctuation, grammar, or vocabulary. The focus is not on how the entries are written, but on what is written.

- It can be helpful to include inspirational notes throughout journal entries. These short reminders can provide added motivation that will stand out as you skim through the pages of the journal.

Reflective Questions for Health Care Providers (write your answers in Part Five):

1) What are some measures that you have your patients take in order to help them heal emotionally and psychologically? What about some measures for their families?

2) What are measures that you take to buoy your psychological and emotional well-being? Have you ever kept a journal for yourself? Why or why not?

3) Have you ever recommended to your patients that they keep a journal to document what they are thinking and feeling as they go through the recovery process? Please explain in detail.

4) Can you list a particular time when you saw or heard about one of your patients benefitting from keeping a journal?

5) If the patient is unable to write, what is an alternative method that you can suggest that might have similar benefits?

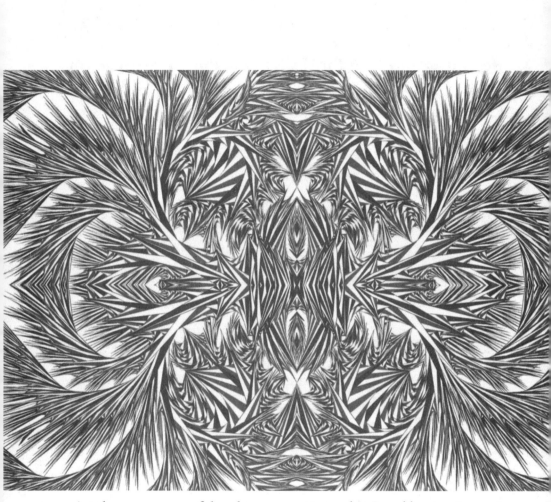

Art therapy was a useful tool to communicate what I could not quite put into words. This large drawing is called *Seizure*, and it took several weeks to complete.

CHAPTER 11

ART THERAPY

Communication can be spoken, gestured through body language, and, as discussed in the previous chapter, written down in a journal. These are powerful forms of communication, but what happens when these three outlets are not available? What if there are things in your mind that you would like to express, but you cannot seem to find the right words to explain exactly what you are thinking and feeling?

To bridge the gap between memories that were spoken and written down in a journal, I would also try to unite these forms into a poem to further describe my experiences.

Deathly tired,
With the setting of the sun.

Panic begins to overwhelm me,
And I lose touch of reality once more.

My mind wanders like a buoy in the sea,
I feel nothing.

A breath of melancholy,
Trembling from nature.

I scream from down deep,
Flaming clouds arise.

The human brain is an extremely powerful tool for processing information from the world that we live in. It also has the ability to create a self-defense mechanism that shields the body from fully experiencing debilitating harm or danger. The mind can quickly shut the body down in traumatic situations, and tragic memories can be repressed, which I have experienced firsthand. In order to effectively treat trauma, we must move beyond the use of words and language so that we can also incorporate the cognitive, emotional, and affective memory (Talwar, 2007).

I do not have a memory of the day of the accident, or the first few days of being in the ICU, but the memory of the eighteen years of my life before the day of the accident is intact. If I piece together all the information that was given to me from my family and friends about what I was doing on the day of the accident, I can sort of imagine doing these activities because they had become a common routine of mine. I cannot truly say how much I vividly remember during the first few days, or even the first few weeks, of being in the hospital, because I was in and out of so many surgeries. My memory is vague from the second that I woke up on July 6, and the concept of time seemed to stop the moment I was flown into shock trauma.

It is a very bizarre experience to not be able to remember certain moments in your life, where several weeks have been transformed into random snippets of a distorted reality. There are entire days for which I cannot account, and this has created a sense of feeling incomplete. I know that I am alive. I can think, feel, hear, and smell, but something is missing.

The only way to explain this sensation is to imagine walking into an art gallery and looking at a painting that is about ten yards away. Upon first glance, it appears to be lacking any colors or shapes; from this distance, the piece looks completely blank, practically disguised by the bright white wall behind it. There are no lines, brushstrokes, or any visible marks from the artist. You can neither confirm nor deny that this empty canvas is blank for a reason, or if the canvas had been painted over. What is the artist trying to say? You wonder if the work is supposed to look like this.

It is not until your eyes are just a few inches from the canvas that you realize there is a masterpiece right in front of you that is made up of very subtle details. The lines, shapes, and visual composition were there all along, practically unseen to the naked eye. The painting existed behind its camouflaged façade, but it existed, just like our memories. Whether we are aware of them or not, or if they are expressed or repressed, sometimes we have to make the attempt to observe, reflect, and then begin the search for what may be hidden.

No matter how much I want to believe that the entire situation was just a nightmare, the scars left behind are very real. To know if I was conscious or unconscious at the accident scene was a certain detail of July 6 that was of great importance to me when I left the hospital. I had several long conversations with my EMS providers over time, and they explained that I was conscious and coherent at the accident scene. Based on my responses to their questions and commands, I had understood what was taking place at the accident scene. They explained that I may have been in an altered state of mind, on the verge of going into shock, but I was aware of my situation. My care providers gave a similar answer about my state during the first couple of days in the hospital.

No matter how hard I have tried, I still cannot recall these events. Would I ever remember these traumatic events? I repeatedly asked my doctors, and the answer was startling—at any time, these hidden memories had the potential of vividly returning. I could be awake or asleep and these experiences could be relived, flashed across my consciousness in real time.

I started to feel some closure when I began communicating to others and to myself about the entire recovery process, by openly talking about my experiences of being in the hospital, writing my thoughts down in a journal, and creating artwork to connect the disconnected fragments of my past. As time went on, I realized that I may not be able to get these memories back, but I could gradually arrange these past experiences into a new stream of memories that would effectively fill in the missing details in a realistic and therapeutic way. It became a way of "tricking" my mind through talking, writing, and creating art about my experiences of going through the recovery process. It was often through artwork that I was able to find the most suitable medium of self-expression when it came to dealing with some of my incomprehensible experiences.

Ever since I was little, I always enjoyed drawing pictures and working on various art projects. I tapped into this hobby again when I was strong enough to skillfully draw while sitting upright. Not only was drawing good for the psychological healing process, but it was also a way for me to strengthen the muscles and nerves in my hands, forearms, and lower back. Having the ability to artistically put my thoughts and memories down on paper was therapeutic for many reasons, but especially because it allowed me to embark on an internal quest in search of understanding my past memories. Once I located these memories, I was able to process these traumatic events and integrate them into my life history (Pifalo, 2007).

I was not quite sure where to start, so I drew lines and random shapes for an extended period of time. Some of my first few projects were very abstract, and I would spend days drawing lines, especially with the colors red, white, and black. I do not know why I chose these colors to work with, but I felt like I was being guided by instinct. I also was not sure where I was going with this type of abstract composition, but it was my way of scratching the surface of the memories trapped within.

I continued with the exploration, similar to the process archaeologists take when they stand over a piece of earth that potentially holds a historically significant artifact. They carefully scrape away at the dirt, looking for clues, reacting to pieces of the mysterious object until it is finally unveiled. Like the archaeologist, I kept digging further into my memories. Over time, these random shapes that were made up of continuous lines evolved into representative imagery.

The intense concentration that took place while illustrating the subject matter helped me focus on the subconscious memories that lay beneath the surface of my mind. What started out as abstract developed into more realistic depictions with surrealistic attributes.

Most of my content was based on recreating scenes of being in a coma, or the hallucinations that I had from the heavy medication. I also explored the limited line of sight that I had as a patient, along with the experience of waking up after the operations, the scenarios that unfolded during the day of the accident, the near-fatal collision, the numerous CAT scans, and the dismal atmosphere that made up my reality.

To illustrate these various scenes, I would often use symbolic colors and imagery that included disorienting compositions of blurred first-person perspectives that would recreate the memories. This is what makes art therapy so extraordinary—an image that appears to be a blotch of colors to someone else is actually a highly detailed expression of how I interpreted my recovery process.

When I began a new project, I rarely had a starting place or final product in mind. The initial goal was to start drawing, and it would lead to an exploration of the haunting and fascinating visions of my past. After I made the first mark on the paper, I would be instantly flooded with memories that were visual representations of my subconscious. My aim was to confront these images through art in order to fully comprehend them and then eventually accept them as a part of my past. During my time in the ICU, my thoughts were often colliding with the living nightmare that I found myself trapped in. It became a challenge to decipher what was actually taking place versus the chemically induced visions I had in the coma, which I explored in drawings, but also paintings, photography, and short film.

When you are comatose, you are neither living nor dead. The physical state of your body is dependent on the pumps and beeps of alien medical equipment. Every time your heart struggles to contract, an artificial beep emanates from the cardiorespiratory machine that sits next to your hospital bed. You wait for that next beep and usually it comes, but when it does not, the machine rapidly sounds an alarm and the care team pumps life into your fragile body. Hopefully, the vital signs return to normal, but normal never lasts and the process is often repeated. This is the routine, day in and day out, and my art tried to convey what this routine was like.

This work of art is a visual narrative of some of my memories from the hospital. I wanted to focus on the randomness of my surroundings

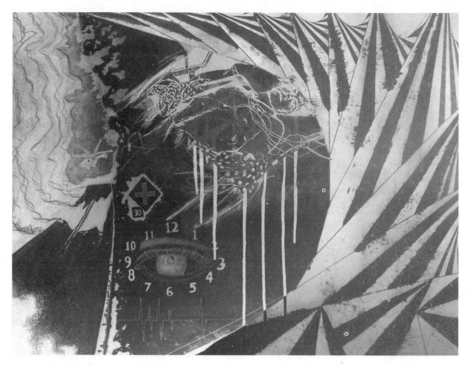

Brian Boyle, *Time is of the Essence,* **2006, graphic pen and charcoal on paper, 24 x 36 in.**

throughout different states of consciousness. The scattered placement of images in the overall composition is meant to represent how, in a comatose state, the body seems to hover without any real order or position. There is no sense of time when you are comatose. The chronological order in which things usually take place is completely absent and random occurrences become the new pattern.

To gain an understanding of the duration of time when my life was on standby, I incorporated some of the various events that I could recall while being comatose. Starting with the foundation of the overall composition, the first thing that I created was the cross on the intersection sign that contrasts with the harsh background. The symbol is a reference to the road sign from the intersection where my accident occurred, which connects with the cross on the helicopter that ominously lingers over the accident scene; the extremely small cross on the floating helicopter also establishes a religious significance. The placement of the eye within the clock is a reference to the time lost while in a coma, and the eye relates both to the watchful surveillance of my family, friends, and care providers as they patiently wait for a sign of survival as well as to my visual perspective of the world revolving around me while I remain stationary, fixated on the blur of my surroundings. The vital sign below the eye clock shows the viewer that life still exists through the pulse, which is further represented by a strong will to live that is constantly being tested throughout the entire journey back to life.

Before I discovered the psychological power of art therapy, I would wake up most mornings and feel as if I were still the figure in this artistic composition, trapped in an inescapable mental prison and paralyzed on the hospital bed in room 19. Every time I look at this specific drawing, I discover something new about what these images represent, which allows even more understanding and healing to take place. This artistic composition is more than a symbol of coming back to life; it represents a tragic memory that I have come to understand better over the years. I may not be able to fully remember all the details of July 6, but my art therapy was an important factor that helped with the healing.

Art therapy is a very effective way to explore the psychological components of our conscious and subconscious. We are able to take the focus away from the self and project it onto the artwork, which allows the artist to fulfill the need for stability and control. Through this visual realm, similar to writing in a journal, we are able to confront our past and take a step closer to understanding and overcoming our traumatic backgrounds and tragic memories.

Suggestions for Health Care Providers and/or Patient's Family:

- Art is a very personal form of self-expression; I suggest the best place to start is with a blank canvas.

- After you start drawing a line or a shape, react to it. How does it make you feel? What does it remind you of? Let your mind roam and wander through your past, present, and future. Visually explore your hopes, fears, dreams, nightmares, worries, goals, and concerns.

- Choose whatever medium you have an interest in: drawing, painting, sculpture, photography, digital video, etc.

- Always keep in mind that this is your work of art, and you are free to create anything you would like. If you like the color blue, add as much blue in the piece as you like. If you like portraits, draw a portrait. If you prefer an Impressionist approach over more of an Abstract method, by all means, go for it.

- Remember that there are no rules or restrictions when it comes to your work. If you want to add a detail or take it out, this is completely up to you.

- The focus should be more on expression than perfection. Go with your instincts and base your decisions on how you are reacting to your art.

Reflective Questions for Health Care Providers (write your answers in Part Five):

1) Do you personally feel that art therapy is effective? Please explain in detail.

2) If you do feel that art therapy is effective, do you recommend it to patients who you think could benefit from it? Why?

3) Can you list a particular time when you saw one of your patients benefit from using art as a part of his or her therapy?

4) Outside of writing in a journal, talking about their experiences, and using art therapy, what other measures do you think patients can take in order to help them cope with the stress they are going through?

5) What types of factors in patients' behavior and outlook would you look for when thinking about incorporating art therapy into their treatment plan?

PART FOUR

COMPASSION

"They may forget your name, but they will never forget how you made them feel."

—Maya Angelou

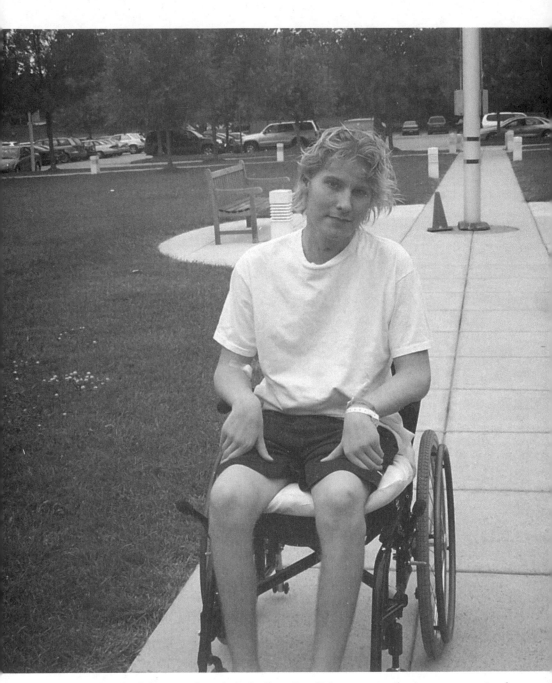

In my wheelchair at the rehab facility; I still have a very long way to go in the recovery process.

CHAPTER 12

SEEING THE WORLD THROUGH THE EYES OF THE PATIENT

You become a patient the moment you are admitted to the hospital. Depending on the size of the hospital, you have become part of a large community governed by the day-in and day-out goings-on in a lifesaving and life-giving atmosphere.

Compassion came from all sources. Because we were in the hospital for so long, we came to know everyone, from the president of the hospital and his staff to the cafeteria group, parking lot attendants, security officers, maintenance workers, and hospital employees from many departments. Our doctors and nurses showed a great sense of compassion and their emotions visually projected their sincerity, sometimes with a tear.

I have learned that the people around you within the health care atmosphere become a new kind of support system, even a new family, that understands the pain and frustration you feel. This new family is not linked by genetics, but rather through life experience.

As a former patient, I know that doctors and nurses share experiences with their coworkers, faculty and staff, and administration. With each day, through a smile or a handshake, a bond forms that develops into friendship, which then leads to a sense of teamwork, and ultimately a sense of accomplishment when various goals are achieved. In this atmosphere, everyone depends on others for help and assistance.

Care providers have a truly extraordinary power. On a daily basis they are not only caring for the health of their patients, they are creating reasons to smile, making living conditions suitable and pleasant, and forming connections with people who not only need them, but put their very lives in their hands.

At a young age I found out what it really means to depend on others. At eighteen, I was not living the normal life of a high school graduate. Instead, I was practically reborn. I had to relearn how to blink, move my fingers, talk, eat, tie my shoes, shower, and do everything in my power to live independently again. I wanted to return to at least somewhat close to the way things were before the accident; that took a lot of help from those around me.

During my coma, there were several times when I overheard my medical team talking about the need to transfer me to a nursing home for twenty-four-hour care the rest of my life. I could not believe that any of this was happening to me. On July 6, all my visions of the future had been crushed. Even though my bones were slowly healing over time, there was no guarantee that my future would ever mend.

It was a horrifying experience, especially when I looked out my room and I saw nurses pushing stretchers by with white sheets covering the other patients because they were not as lucky as me. As frightened as I became from looking out into the ICU, I also became an object that frightened those who passed by my room.

One memory I will never forget is when a mother and her daughter stopped by my open door to talk to a nurse who was sitting outside my room. The little girl hesitantly looked into my room, and then her eyes widened and she screamed, "Mommy, there's a monster in that room!" The woman, confused, glanced at me and then quickly put her hand over her daughter's eyes to shield her from looking at me, stating, "Oh, good Lord, honey, don't look at that!"

She grabbed her daughter and rushed off, and I sank in absolute shame, as if I were no longer human. Did I really look that bad? I was so ashamed of what I had become—nothing more than a science experiment with wires and tubes interwoven throughout my body. As hurt as I was by the little girl's reaction, I did not blame her. If I had happened to see my reflection in the mirror, I too would have been shocked and frightened.

I remember my parents coming into my room several times a day, and they would stand there and desperately beg me to stay strong and keep fighting, while also trying to explain to me the situation that I was in. With all the sadness that we were facing as a family, there were still some good things happening, even though they rarely occurred during this stage.

One of those amazing days came when I was able to learn how to talk again—a day my parents and I will never forget. After several attempts to get me to say a few syllables, one lucky day, it just happened out of nowhere. My respiratory therapist hooked up a speaking valve to my trach, and I tried to sound out a few words and all of a sudden I began talking. All the nurses and doctors came running in and broke out in tears when they heard me. My parents, who had just arrived, came running around the corner; they were awestruck. I told my dad that everything was going to be okay, and he just burst into tears. As for my mom, I do not think she stopped crying for the entire two months I was there, but at least in that moment, these were finally tears of joy.

It was not only my personal experiences in the hospital that made a permanent impact on me. The memories of the other patients and their families have also been forever woven into the delicate fabric of my living nightmare and my ongoing thoughts.

There was a family that would walk by my room each day around the evening visiting hour session. I would usually see the mother and father, and occasionally there would be two teenage girls with them. This family really stood out to me because the intensely desperate look on their faces was very similar to how my parents looked during the early stages of my recovery when I started to regain consciousness.

I recognized that exhausted and defeated gaze, the tissues near the face, the slumped shoulders, the quiet determination. I didn't know who they were visiting, but I knew they were in the next room. There was always a little hesitation before they walked into the room. They would look inside, then look at the ground, take a deep breath, and move out of my sight to visit their loved one.

One afternoon shortly before I was transferred out of the ICU, my nurse took me outside to get some fresh air. As I sat in my wheelchair a few feet outside my room, waiting to go outside, I was approached by the mother of the family I had become used to seeing on a daily basis. In a trembling voice, she forced a smile and explained that her son was around the same age as me and was in the room adjacent to mine. He had been flown into shock trauma the previous week practically DOA. He had been at a party with some friends and a fight broke out; a verbal argument quickly escalated into violence. Witnesses reported that her son had tried to step in and ameliorate the situation, but unfortunately, one of the people in the altercation took out a gun and shot him, then quickly fled the scene.

Her eyes widened in panic as if she was momentarily imagining what it must have been like to be a bystander in that room. She paused for a bit when reality caught up to her. After she wiped tears from her face, she further explained that there was a lot of damage and he had to be revived several times on the operating table. In extremely critical condition, they were unsure whether he would make it through the next few days.

I looked at her and tried to grasp everything she had told me. I did my best to imagine her pain and also the pain of what my parents had to go through with me. I reflected on their agony and suffering. No matter how hard I tried, I could not even imagine how terrible a feeling it must have been.

She put her hand on my shoulder and told me that my parents had shared a little bit of my background, injuries, and progress with her family in the waiting room, and that had given them so much to believe in. She said that she wanted her little boy back in any way that she could get him back, which is the same statement that I overheard my dad say on the day that they realized I was giving up.

She looked me in the eyes and explained that seeing me in the wheelchair was concrete proof that miracles do happen, and that gave her so much hope that her son could have a similar recovery. She said that talking to me and knowing a little bit about what I had been through had given her so much strength to stay strong for both her son and her family.

For the rest of that day, I remember lying in the hospital bed with my eyes tightly locked on the wall on the right side of the room, envisioning this young man on the opposite side, fighting for his life. His parents and sisters might have been on both sides of his bed, holding his hands, watching his chest rise and fall with every assisted breath. Would he survive? It was uncertain, but his family had to believe that he would. They had to believe that he would make it through the next day.

Every day there were more reminders of how unforgiving life could be to some people. Why do people have to suffer? I was only a teenager, but I was quickly growing up and having to ponder things that do not usually cross the mind of a typical eighteen-year-old guy.

I remember that when I was in and out of the medical facilities, I would look around the room and see people just like me struggling to perform the most basic tasks with their therapists, nurses, and support staff. Full-grown men cried out in pain as they tried to bench-press a broomstick. A young boy learning how to walk again after a drunk driver ran him over. A twelve-year-old girl who had lost her arms and legs to a flesh-eating disease hid her tears behind sunglasses while she tried to learn how to sit up in a chair without falling over.

These are just a handful of memories I will never forget, and I honestly do not want to forget them because they are a part of my life that has made me the person I am.

It was all there—the breathtaking sadness, the human misery, complete despair, and tragic heartbreak. Even with all this hardship, it was still evident that when you took away the catastrophic injuries, or the debilitating disease, or the effects of old age, you found regular people who once lived normal, everyday lives. When you are a patient in a hospital or a rehab center, you witness extraordinary individuals who personify determination in its truest form.

These resilient people do not know what giving up means, and every fiber of their being is intensely focused on making progress in their lives. Most of these people did not have a choice when it came to experiencing these traumas, but they did have a choice to persevere on and deal with the hand they were dealt in life. When it comes to overcoming the odds stacked against them, nothing is ever guaranteed, but everything is earned.

Within each person, whether said or not, the challenge was an internal battle, conducted privately for themselves, but the health care provider played an important part in that battle.

Victory was measured in the smallest increments, like blinking, or moving a finger, but most importantly, victory was achieved—no matter how big or small each achievement—through the work of care providers.

Suggestions for Health Care Providers and/or Patient's Family:

- Try to keep negative stimuli from patients and their families. Remember that visitors are most likely inexperienced and unacquainted with the hospital environment, and the sights and scenes may be alarming to them.
- Try to always be sensitive to the tremendous "battles" patients and their families have fought and will fight in the future.

Reflective Questions for Health Care Providers (write your answers in Part Five):

1) How can you become engaged with your coworkers, patients, and visitors? What are some simple ways you can show people you care?

2) How can you show your commitment to your organization's vision and mission? Do you think your level of commitment will trickle down to your patient care strategy?

3) Try to remember a time when you experienced a small triumph with a patient as he or she accomplished a goal. How did this make you feel?

4) Do you think that having your patients and their families see other patients and their families in similar situations will help them heal and cope? How so?

5) How do you deal with the unfairness (e.g., who lives and who dies) of life and how precarious life can be?

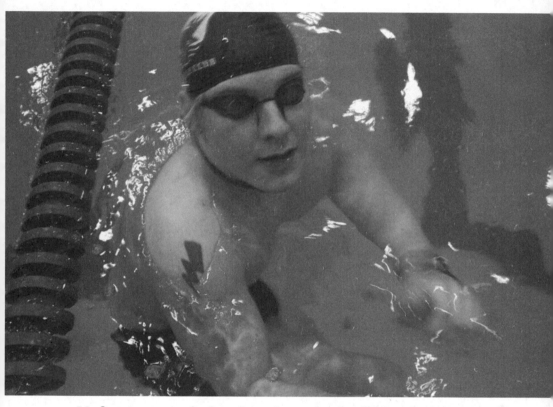

My first time getting back in the pool—six months after leaving the ICU. I used to be a state champion swimmer, and now I could barely stay afloat.

CHAPTER 13

THE GOLDEN RULE

THE ETHIC OF RECIPROCITY, OR THE GOLDEN RULE, IS TO TREAT OTHERS as you would like to be treated. This ethical code spans across many religions and philosophies throughout the world. Although stated differently, the message is the same. It sounds simple enough, but this moral statement can be neglected in our daily lives.

We live and work in an ever-quickening environment, but no matter how busy our schedule is or how fast-paced our world gets, it is critical that we are aware of how we talk to the people we encounter each day, both friends and complete strangers.

I recall a conversation with one of my physical therapists during rehabilitation that has stuck with me to the present day. I was sitting in my wheelchair during one of the initial sessions, and I was discussing with him my hope of being able to get back in the pool as a part of my physical therapy; we chose that specific rehab center because they had a pool and we were told that getting in the pool would be a part of my therapy. I was not trying to swim competitively, but I wanted to be back in the pool again because I knew it would bring peace of mind.

Most of my time during my high school years was spent at the pool. I could be found at the indoor pool from fall to spring, and at the outdoor pool during the summer. Growing up on the swim team, it was just the normal lifestyle.

After leaving the ICU, I was making progress each day. I daydreamed about getting back in the water, to dog-paddle, float, or whatever I was able to do, as long as I could get in the water. Even though I was one hundred pounds lighter, I felt like I weighed two tons because of the amount of muscle and strength I lost while in the coma. I longed for that magical feeling of being weightless, and the pool is where I needed to go.

When I asked the therapist when we could incorporate getting in the pool as a part of my therapy, he gave me a puzzled look. He brushed off what I said and told me that with my background and injuries, getting back in the pool was not a possibility; I was not strong enough to get in the water, and my heart and lungs could not handle the humid air.

I tried to be optimistic. I gave him the benefit of the doubt. Maybe he was right. I would need to let my lungs heal a bit more, because it could be warm in the indoor pool. I was also hopeful that my heart rate would eventually return to normal, as well as my strength. For the moment, I had to direct my thoughts on trying to be patient.

After a minute of convincing myself I had to wait on getting back in the pool, I curiously asked him what he thought my chances were of ever swimming again. With the same puzzled look on his face, he told me it would be best if I considered pursuing a different activity, because swimming was unlikely. Even after the previous weeks of dealing with setbacks and negativity, I did not think I could feel any more defeated. I was wrong.

I was quiet for the rest of that therapy session. Where were the encouraging words? The motivational support? He had just met me and read over my chart; how did he know for sure that I would never be able to swim again? He didn't know me or my work ethic. I just couldn't understand how somebody could be that direct, with complete disregard for the devastating impact of his words.

I tried to view most hurdles that stood in my way throughout recovery as opportunities rather than challenges. I have never been the type of person to have to prove doubters wrong. However, when I was told swimming was an unrealistic goal for me, I seriously reflected on my current situation. Maybe in the moment it was foolish to think about getting back in the pool, but one day things would be different. I had to stay positive and believe that if I worked hard every day, I could restore my muscular and cardiovascular systems. I would work on developing everything back to where it used to be.

When talking with the patient and family, it is very important to be cognizant of not only what you are saying to them regarding their current and future medical treatment, but also *how* you are saying it. They have thoughts, feelings, concerns, and worries, and they are scared and have a lot of questions. You may not be in a position to answer all of their questions, but you can do your part to help them thoroughly understand their situation. This will help establish a strong foundation of trust with the family. You will also be able to help alleviate some of their anxiety through the way that you interact with them.

In one focus group composed of twenty-six nurses regarding their contribution to positive patient experiences, a nurse suggested that "nursing care is about being heard and seen. Knowing that you are in safe hands. You allay their fear and uncertainty. You give patients confidence and hope in return" (Kieft, Brouwer, Francke & Delnoij, 2014, p. 4).

When it comes to the golden rule with your patients and their families, it is important to quickly find a way to relate to them, which is not always an easy task. It is helpful to get on their level and make a connection, because every conversation with them thereafter will be much easier and that trust will be strengthened.

Occasionally, time constraints might not allow for this connection to develop, especially in emergency situations where time is of the essence. Whether you have a few minutes or a few seconds, try to use understandable vocabulary when communicating any type of information to the family. Taking the time to speak to the family is an opportunity to seek further solutions and the appropriate measures that can ultimately help the treatment of the patient.

Keep in mind that the family is going to be perceptive of every word that you say. If you state that something is going to improve or decline with the patient's progress, they are going to hold you accountable. If the patient is in critical condition, the thought of dying is always in the back of the family's mind. They do not want to think the worst, but they know that there is a possibility where progress might not take place and death might be inevitable.

If you have to convey bad news or tell a family that their loved one has passed or is going to pass, it is important to present the information in a calm manner and explain that your team is doing all they can to help improve the health of the patient. It is appropriate to be realistic but also to present the information in a way where the tone is not overly negative. My care providers had a special way of answering questions without giving too many distressing details. It worked well.

In his book, *M.D.: Doctors Talk about Themselves*, Dr. John Pekkanen explains his method of giving bad news to his medical students: "I teach them to tell patients that some people with their illness live for only a few months, but others can survive for several years, and there is no way to predict how you will do."

In such situations, explain the details as if you were having to tell this to a close friend. You can address any concerns or questions they may have. Even if you cannot provide feedback on every question, take the time to hear their concerns, because it shows them that you care about their loved one.

Suggestions for Health Care Providers and/or Patient's Family:

- Speak in a gentle tone of voice. Use the family's names and the name of the patient frequently; this shows them that you are acknowledging their family and their loved one.
- Use uplifting words and phrases as often as possible, because they will create a positive atmosphere.
- Try to form a connection with patients and families to establish a sense of trust before you give them any medical updates.
- Reflect on the type of family you are talking to, and present the information in a compassionate way rather than just stating the facts.
- Provide realistic expectations that they should have regarding treatment and progress.

Reflective Questions for Health Care Providers (write your answers in Part Five):

1) If you were the family member, what would you like to hear in order to help alleviate pain as the reality of the situation sets in? What are things that you would not like to hear?
2) In your experiences as a care provider, what are specific measures that you have taken to connect with a patient and his or her

family? Which measures worked best, and which measures did not work at all?

3) What can you say to the family about what you are doing for the patient without giving false promises? (E.g., "We are doing all that we can, but we have to wait and see.")

4) How can you encourage your patient to realize that even small goals matter?

5) How can you encourage the family of the patient to appreciate that even small improvements are monumental events taking place?

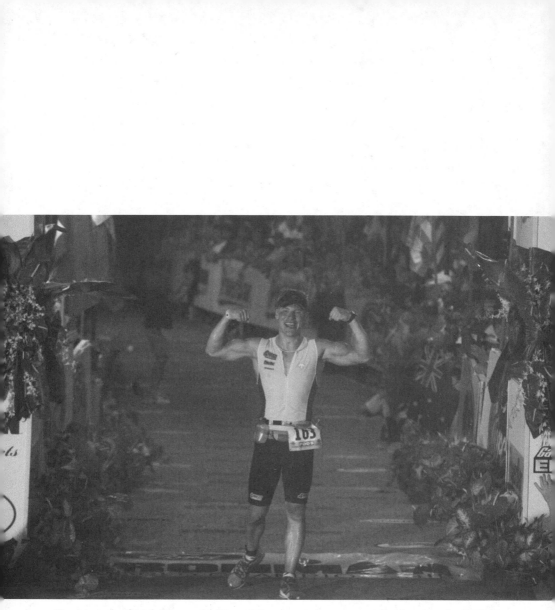

Crossing the finish line at the Hawaii Ironman, three years after leaving the ICU. A sense of closure had been achieved and my recovery was finally complete.

CHAPTER 14

THE STAGES OF GRIEF

W ITHIN THE FIRST FEW MINUTES OF A CONVERSATION, YOU CAN USUALLY gain a sense of someone's personality, background, and whether he or she prefers to hear all the facts or just a quick summary of the details. You can acquire this knowledge from the patient and his or her family by having a small conversation with them to briefly get to know them, which can be helpful when explaining the routine ups and downs of the patient's progress.

Some topics are not easy to broach, especially with a patient or family you already know tends to be emotional and on edge. In situations where their frustration turns to anger, please understand that this reaction is directed at the situation and not at you personally, even though you may feel like it sometimes. You are the one who must give them disheartening and tragic news, which is never easy. They may feel that because you are explaining the circumstances to them, you also have the power to make things better regarding their loved one's health.

When you have to tell the family that their loved one has passed away or is not going to survive much longer, the family begins going through the five stages of grief that Elisabeth Kübler-Ross introduces in her book

On Death and Dying. (I know that many people are familiar with this concept, but I would like to share suggestions based on my family's experience.) The first stage is denial. The family has an initial tendency not to accept the tragic reality and may psychologically alter the circumstances in their minds to make it more tolerable. They are in a very desperate state at this moment and will transition to the next stage—anger—when they realize they can no longer deny the inevitable. Showing anger is common because the information is too unbearable to comprehend, and it overloads their understanding of why things happened the way they did.

If they believe in a higher power, they will begin offering promises in the bargaining stage in order to prolong the life of their loved one. Even after death has been declared, some family members will plead with care providers to go back into the unit and work until their loved one comes back to life.

Throughout the first three stages, please do not get discouraged. You can do only so much as the care provider, and the family has to realize this. They usually do after the information starts to settle into their tormented consciousness. They have entered the stage of depression at this point, which can be a long and difficult process full of tears, regret, and detachment from those closest to them, because their view of life has been defeated on many levels.

Over time, as they come to absorb the unfortunate reality, they will also accept the circumstances. Their emotional and psychological wounds will have healed and their outlook on life will become more stable compared to how it was during the previous stages.

Every individual, family, and situation will be different. I believe that people react to things based on their pre-existing views and life experiences. There are people who will race through these five stages of grief; others will go back and forth between the stages. Some will exist in a state of depression for a very long time, and the loss in their heart will never truly be healed. From my personal experience and the people I have met over the years, I have learned that there are some individuals who never reach a full sense of closure.

When you walk into an ICU waiting room, you get an up-close look at people going through the various stages of grief. It is never an easy experience watching others suffer, but it is a daily occurrence in this setting. Families congregate in the waiting room after they finish visiting their loved ones. Not long after they enter this room, the reality of what they just saw starts to hit them like a ton of bricks. My parents talk about how some of the visitors would sit there, completely in shock, with their bodies frozen like statues. Other visitors would pace around the room in frustration, some people would get angry out of complete desperation, and some would hysterically cry for hours. Everyone had a different way of experiencing grief.

My parents saw other families go through the same motions. Some families were there for short-term patients, and some, like my family, were there long term. My parents explained to me that over time there would be friendly interactions that took place with the people you saw on a frequent basis. You reached out to others, while others did the same. After a while, you got to know their family, learn about their loved one in the hospital, and become familiar with their entire experience. Just like in the hospital room, there was a system of support among the families in the waiting room. Effective coping strategies were exchanged and pursued.

The waiting room becomes a place where a lot of big decisions have to be made. Families are confronted with life-and-death situations that are changing every minute. However, every minute spent in the waiting room is a good sign because that is another minute that their loved one is still living.

Suggestions for Health Care Providers and/or Patient's Family:

- When dealing with the grief of the patient and his or her family, offer reassurance and support.
- Try to remember and recognize all the stages of grief.
- Remember not to take things personally when a family is distraught.
- As a care provider, remember that you are the biggest ally for the family and that you have the power to help guide them through the recovery process, both the ups and the downs.

Reflective Questions for Health Care Providers (write your answers in Part Five):

1) How did you feel the first time you observed a patient's loved ones going through the various stages of grief? How do you feel now when you see it?

2) How do you prepare yourself before you have to give bad news to a patient or a patient's family member?

3) When you do have to present bad news to a patient or family, do you feel that you disconnect from the situation to help get you through the conversation? What helps you mentally recover after you give bad news?

4) Is there anything you have noticed over the years that has helped the family reach a sense of closure?

5) What is a measure that you take with the patient's loved ones when they refuse to accept bad news and take the frustration out on you? Please explain.

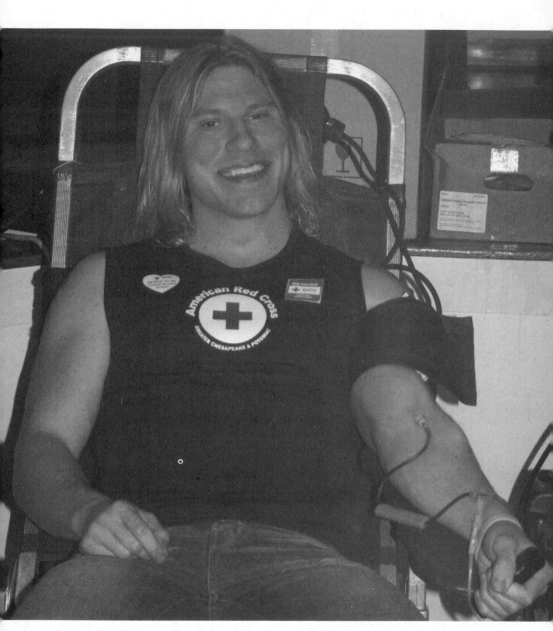

I wanted to live up to the promise I made to myself when I was at the rehab center, so I became a Red Cross volunteer and donated blood at the hospital that saved my life.

CHAPTER 15

WHY DO SOME PATIENTS HEAL, WHILE OTHERS DO NOT?

In the summer of 2004, I remember lying in my hospital bed and trying my best to be positive. It was not easy when I looked at what was left of me: a body covered in tangled wires and tubes, IVs piercing my flesh from head to toe, and electricity and blood keeping my heart beating.

As a long-term patient in the ICU, it was a very disorienting environment to "wake up" in every day, because I could not tell what I was waking up to. How long had I been asleep since the last time I was aware? Did a few hours go by, or was it more like days? It felt like I was living a nightmare. It was truly frightening.

During the day I went back and forth between sensory deprivation and sensory overload. There was a fine line between these two states, but no matter where I found myself, my mind was in a fog. I tried to block the noises out, but in a place like the ICU, peace and quiet do not exist. The constant beeping, alarms, and noises from the machines next to my hospital bed were not there for decoration. As much as I wanted the noise to stop, I knew that each beep and buzz from that equipment was audible proof that I was still on this planet. The depressing atmosphere was taking a heavy toll on me, and I could not escape it.

The pain I was experiencing was beyond words, but what really did me in was not the pain from my injuries but seeing my parents suffer every time they walked into my room. The love from my family kept me going, but my will to continue on was slowly starting to erode. I did not want to live the rest of my life in a hospital bed in a nursing home. As this started to become what my future would look like, I contemplated giving up. My heart swells just reflecting on that period. Life had become too much for me to bear, and I felt I had only one choice at the time. This was the lowest point in my life. I had hit rock bottom.

One morning, when I heard the nurses discussing the possibility of transferring me to a long-term-care nursing home, I made my final decision. I was not proud of it, but I did not see any alternative. I gave up my attempt at any communication, I no longer responded to any commands, and I lay there trying to find the peace I was seeking. I had escaped the grasp of death several times already during my recovery, but this time, I would not attempt to overcome it.

I simply lay there on my back, thinking about times and places much happier than room 19. I thought about my family, my friends, the goals that I had set out for myself, what I had already accomplished, and the way things would be when I was gone. My eyes burned as tears began streaming down my paralyzed face.

Later that afternoon, my parents arrived for visiting hours. As I mentioned in an earlier chapter about the special power that parents have when it comes to their children, my parents somehow knew what was going through my mind and what I had decided to do. I realized this because they acted differently from the dozens of times I had seen them before. My dad knew that now was the time he had to plead with me not to give up. My mom was standing near him, and my dad was raising his voice to let me know how serious the situation was. He begged me to stay strong, for myself, for them, for my friends, and for my future wife and children. I had to keep going. He told me that we were almost out of the woods, and very soon things would be so much different, but I had to make the decision to keep going, to keep clawing my way back to the living.

It was a very emotional experience, and after my dad finished talking, he practically collapsed onto the aqua-colored chair near my bed, physically and emotionally exhausted.

As minutes ticked by, I focused my thoughts on when human suffering finally ends—when the body dies and the human spirit takes over. My mom and my dad were not going to let me die, and I realized that in that moment, on top of all the machines that had been keeping me alive, it was their love that was going to save me from this darkness. I made a new decision: I was not going to die in that hospital bed or in a nursing home. I was going to survive and get my life back again. I realized that all of my goals and dreams may have been shattered just like the bones in my body, but bones can be mended. So can dreams.

I began to focus my energy and strength on redeveloping the muscles in my face so I could smile for my parents. Just a few hours after the last-resort talk that my dad had with me, I gave him and my mother a smile. This subtle expression was a visual clue to my parents that I was still there for them and fighting to escape the looming grip of death.

I did everything in my own power to improve and crawl my way back to the living. I moved my toes to get my feet to move. I chewed ice to learn how to eat. I went through a long and agonizing process to learn how to talk. I look back at all these events now, and they seem so small and easy, but back then they were monumental breakthroughs on my road to recovery.

I kept focusing my attention on accomplishing these tasks, taking baby steps to go on to the next one and then the next, but I continued to reach for progress. The joy that it brought to the faces of my family and friends inspired me to keep pushing for further improvement. I was so used to seeing everyone with tears in their eyes, but I finally began seeing tears of joy and it meant the world to me.

Several weeks slowly went by, and instead of doing what all my friends in college were doing, I was being transferred to a rehabilitation center. While there, I continued the process of learning how to talk, eat, tie my shoes, shower, and live independently again, at least somewhat close to the way things used to be—with a lot of help from those around me.

Even with all my progress, I still was not really sure what my future would consist of. At the time, I was just happy to be alive and out of the hospital, but in the back of my mind something was pushing me to see how far I could go. I thought of all the limitations that were placed on me and all the medical problems I was diagnosed with, and I used that as my motivation. I had to prove to myself that I was not going to let this tragedy stop me from pursuing what I had originally planned for my life.

I have always been fascinated by what inspires us during times of great adversity. Is it past experience, support from a friend or a loved one, or future goals that we are striving to accomplish? I personally feel that our motivation can be based on a combination of all of the above, which helps us become more resilient.

In the book *Resilience: Discovering a New Strength at Times of Stress*, Frederic Flach explains that "resilience depends on our ability to recognize pain, acknowledge its purpose, tolerate it for a reasonable time until things begin to take shape, and resolve our conflicts constructively." We begin the healing process once we recognize the pain that we are experiencing, and it is then that we can overcome the pain and suffering.

I tried my best to be resilient, and it was not easy. After several months of physical therapy, I was able to attend college and participate on the swim team a year after leaving the ICU. Two years later, another goal was realized when I had the chance to compete in the Hawaii Ironman. During the triathlon, when my blood was pumping and my heart was racing, I thought about how they were once signs that I was dying, and now they were signs that I was living. Quitting was never an option during the race. I finished because at one point in time I had given up in the hospital and after I fought back from that very sad moment I made a promise to myself that I would never quit anything ever again. It was the love and support from my family and friends that helped me get to the finish line.

I have learned that no matter what life throws at you, you have the strength within you to overcome it, and with the right attitude you can achieve anything you set your mind to. Life is a series of constant challenges, and you have to be ready and willing to do everything in your power to move forward through all the hardship, obstacles, and negativity. Through this, you will find success.

Live life to the fullest. Set your mind and heart on as many endeavors as possible because you can never have too much on your plate—even though there will be those who look at you and doubt what you are able to do. Do not listen to them. Deep down you know what you are truly capable of. Within you are the capabilities to set goals and to achieve them. Never limit yourself and remember that when other people say something is impossible, that is just their opinion.

The path you are on now may be a different path a year from now. It is normal to change this path once or even several times before you finally decide what you would like to do, and, better yet, what you are *meant* to do.

Life is really what you choose to make of it. The more you sacrifice and invest, the more you will get in return. In order to achieve great things you must be willing to take big risks, depending on what the task is. Life is a complete mystery. All you have is the present and tomorrow is not guaranteed. I find it is very important to focus on what you do have rather than what you do not.

We all have our own experiences in life that have made us who we are. You do not have to be in a coma or in intensive care for two months to understand life any better than someone else. Herodotus, the Greek philosopher, said, "Adversity has the effect of drawing out strength and qualities of a man that would have lain dormant in its absence." Every day we all face our own moments of adversity, both large and small, and we are tested. We do the best we can with what we have.

But just like anything else, there will always be obstacles out there, and it is how we go about facing these obstacles that will make the difference. Having character traits that include honesty, determination, and responsibility will help make a positive outcome.

I truly believe that it is through our observation of those around us that we develop these traits of character—through our parents, family, role models, teachers, and friends. They set the example and prepare us for the present and the future. In order to be honest, we must be truthful through our words and actions. In order for us to show determination, we must persevere through the obstacles in our path. In order to be responsible, we must take ownership of our decisions. Ultimately, in order to learn, we must act.

As Aristotle notes in his *Nicomachean Ethics*, "For the things we have to learn before we can do them, we learn by doing them; e.g., men become builders by building and lyre players by playing the lyre; so too we become just by doing just acts, temperate by doing temperate acts, brave by doing brave acts." Our character traits and abilities are reflected and defined through the experiences that we each face on a daily basis; therefore, they define who we are over time.

When it comes down to why some people heal and others do not, I cannot speak for everybody. But, from my experience, I could have just as easily given up in my hospital bed or gone down a path of clinical depression after leaving the hospital if I did not have such an encouraging support system and a positive attitude. I had many rough moments in the hospital, but I focused on staying optimistic and approaching each challenge as an opportunity for continued healing and personal growth.

I met a lot of very resilient people throughout the recovery process. One outstanding individual was a middle-aged man named Gerry whom I met at the rehab center. He was paralyzed and had been in the facility for several weeks because his medical team was trying a type of new procedure to fix his broken back. He navigated around with the aid of a wheelchair, and one day when I was taking a break from my physical therapy he wheeled himself over and asked how I was doing. During our conversation I learned that he too had been in a motor vehicle accident, and his brother, mother, wife, and daughter were killed. Gerry was the only survivor and my heart ached for him. No matter how hard I tried, I could not even come close to imagining the pain he was going through. Yet he had a presence to him, an energy. I would see him throughout the day during our physical and occupational therapy sessions, and he would go around the room and do his part to motivate the other patients in the unit, including me.

On the day that I left the rehab center, Gerry and his physical therapist approached my parents and me in the long hallway near the exit of the facility. He told me that he wanted to show me something before I left. His physical therapist cautiously stood beside his wheelchair as he slowly lifted his feet down onto the tiled floor. He paused to catch his breath, carefully scooted forward a few inches, and used every bit of his strength to stand up on his own two feet. My parents and I looked at him in amazement as he started taking a few small steps toward us so he could shake my hand and say good-bye. I remember looking up at him from my wheelchair and thinking to myself that this man just lost his family in a tragedy, he would be going home soon to an empty house, but his life was not over. This memory will always be etched in my heart because in that moment Gerry was showing me what it meant to be resilient—not only to survive, but to thrive.

When a challenge is presented to us, as a patient or care provider, we do our best to overcome whatever the situation is. As a result, we learn something about ourselves that makes us stronger. We acknowledge that our mistakes can be learning opportunities. A tragedy can be transformed into a triumph, and an obstacle can be the gateway to success.

Suggestions for Health Care Providers and/or Patient's Family:

- Do not take a single second for granted.
- Take the time out of your day to tell those close to you that you love them.
- Smile more and frown less.
- Show gratitude.
- Perform random acts of kindness for friends and strangers.

- Do not hold grudges.
- Be thankful for what you have and the problems that you do not have.
- Volunteer for a cause that you believe in.
- Get out of your comfort zone every once in a while and try something new.
- Be positive and optimistic.
- Go for a long walk to breathe in the life all around you.
- Make every step, every heartbeat, every moment, and every day count.

Reflective Questions for Health Care Providers (write your answers in Part Five):

1) What are three things that you can do today to show somebody in your life that you think he or she is special?
2) Identify a time when you can recall feeling down and another person helped you.
3) Who inspires and motivates you? Why?
4) How does the work that you do help contribute to making society a better place?
5) Can you think of possible ways to encourage patients who seem to have lost their motivation? List some.

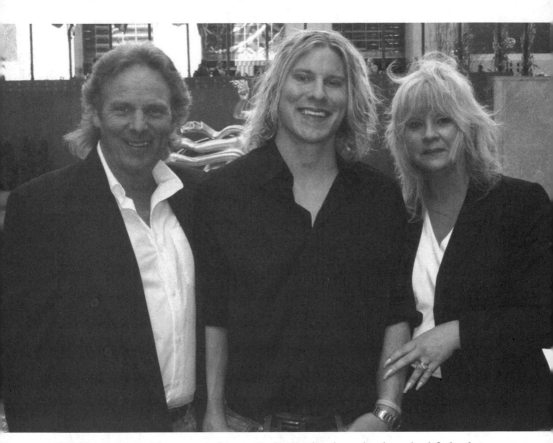

Health care providers not only save individuals, they also breathe life back into families. My care team took care of my parents so they could take care of me, and their strength gave me strength in times when I desperately needed it.

CHAPTER 16

AVOIDING BURNOUT SYNDROME

Throughout the three years that it took to complete the healing process, I was transported to many hospitals and rehabilitation centers that specialized in certain phases of my recovery—shock trauma, ICU, emergency, cardiology, rehabilitation, and outpatient.

Looking through my medical records—stacked over a foot high with folders and loose sheets of paper—I calculated that I had around four dozen care providers whom I remember treating me. This does not even include the many people working behind the scenes to keep me alive and stable.

Every once and a great while, I would meet one of my health care providers who I felt had become hardened or burned out from working in the hospital. In the book *What to Do When Someone You Love Is Depressed: A Practical, Compassionate, and Helpful Guide*, Mitch and Susan Golant explain that "burnout, also called compassion fatigue, is the feeling of having reached the limits of your endurance and your ability to cope." The men and women who I thought were experiencing burnout represented a variety of ages and came from all backgrounds in the health profession, and they all shared a similar unenthusiastic demeanor. They rarely smiled, laughed, pursued conversation, or showed any sign of sincere compassion. When they walked into my room, they would not engage with me. They would do what they had to do to help treat me and alleviate any pain, and they were good at what they did, but there was an obvious disconnect.

Having an empathetic bedside manner was not a top priority to them, but as the patient, it was important to me, and to my parents. It was as if they were focused only on treating the body, rather than the whole person. I wondered if they were always like this or if there was something that led to this type of personality shortcoming?

There were a few veteran health care staff who had been in the system for decades that fit this description, but this was not always the case. I interacted with brand-new health professionals, who, within a single year on the job, had already built walls that prevented them from tending to the human factors involved in healing.

I do not work in the health care system, nor do I know what it is like to care for sick patients on a daily basis. I did not go to school to study medicine, nursing, physical and occupational therapy, etc. I do not know what it is like to lose a patient, to hold his or her hand when that patient takes his or her last breath. However, I do know what it is like to be the patient at death's door, where every steady beat of the heart is considered tremendous progress.

From the moment I was brought into the hospital, I was helpless in a lot of ways and dependent on every single person around me not only to take care of me, but to comfort me. I was more than just flesh, bone, and blood being treated and operated on. I was a person who had a loving family and supportive friends. I had a life before all this happened to me, a future with hopes and dreams.

I am not going to offer a specific method to avoid burnout while working in a hospital. There is no exact science to keep this from happening. Honestly, I can see how this might happen over time when you are dealing with a constant cycle of patients who face life-and-death situations. Depending on the department of the hospital you work in, these life-and-death scenarios can occur daily, and often do.

You may work a twelve-hour shift, but when you leave the hospital to go home, that does not always mean you are done with work; thoughts of your patients are always on your mind. You carry them psychologically with you wherever you go; you could be going to the grocery store and all of a sudden a memory of your patient flashes through your mind. *Is he or she doing okay? Have I done everything in my power to help my patient? What will tomorrow be like for him or her? How can I do my part to improve my patient's quality of life?* These are constant reminders that you cannot just switch off from your work at the end of the day like with other jobs.

There is nothing easy about working in the hospital. From my view of the world, I realized men and women who wear scrubs and white lab coats are not just people doing their job, but real-life superheroes doing their part to make the world a better place. Every one of these life-giving superheroes was brought into the field of health care for a reason. They had a crystal-clear vision of their future, where they would be in a position to help others.

In a study conducted by Geiger-Brown et al. (2012), the sleep patterns of eighty full-time (≥36 h/wk) nurses were analyzed to measure their performance and fatigue levels. The main finding of the study concluded, "Working successive twelve-hour work shifts achieves an inadequate amount of sleep between shifts to recover physically or cognitively, irrespective of whether they work the day or the night shift. Nurses experienced greater sleepiness by their third consecutive twelve-hour shift." The busy schedule of care providers is only one factor that can result in physical and emotional fatigue.

In some cases where I found that it might be necessary, I wanted to return the favor by helping some of my care providers who I thought could use a little motivational boost. Even people who are in the profession of caring for others need to be cared for every once in a while. When I met one of my care providers who I felt had become hardened or desensitized, I made it my personal goal to break the shell he or she had formed. It was a work in progress, just like everything else, and I knew it would not happen within a few hours or a few days. I was a long-term patient so I had all the time in the world, and I wanted to do my part by helping them as they had been helping me. I kept chipping away with a smile, a wave, a grateful acknowledgment of what they were doing. As weak as I was, I wanted to show progress because I could see how much joy it brought them.

When I learned how to talk again, I would talk with them and get to know their background and lifestyle; I could slowly see that they were letting their guard down. I did everything in my limited strength to let them know how special I thought they were and how much I appreciated all they were doing not only to save me, but to save my family.

Not all patients and their families will be grateful for what you are doing, but you have to keep in mind that most of the patients and families will be grateful, even if they do not express it verbally. You take the good with the bad, and focus on the best to help improve the situation.

I am not suggesting that every care provider should have a personality similar to Robin Williams in the movie *Patch Adams*, but what I am requesting is that when there are moments throughout the day when you feel overwhelmed or discouraged, take a second to remember why you wanted to get involved in health care in the first place. What inspired you to enter this field? There is a reason that motivated you to pursue this path, and it is crucial to always reflect on that reason.

Being a care provider is not a job; it is a passion, a calling. You give so much of yourself on a daily basis and your selfless goal is to allevi-

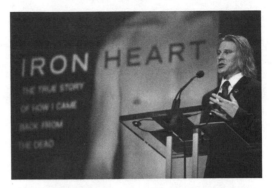

When I learned how to talk again in the hospital, I soon realized that the power of the voice is amplified when the message is one of gratitude.

ate the pain and suffering of your patients and their families. Not everyone will react the same to dealing with somebody who is in pain. People have different strategies to handle the daily stress that comes from working in this field—you see a lot of life-and-death scenarios and people who are experiencing the lowest point in their lives.

The world can be beautiful one second and turn tragic the next. I completely understand that some people do not want to spend a lot of time making a connection with their patients. The schedule is busy, and there are a dozen other patients to look after. You might not want to establish a bond because you would rather keep the relationship distant. Perhaps it is a very serious case, and the priority is keeping the patient alive. It is okay to shield your emotions and disconnect your sensitivity in the hospital, because the job can take a heavy toll when you lose a patient that you have established a strong connection with. In the moment, your full focus is on treating the injury or illness. However, when you walk into a patient's room, please do not forget that you are interacting with a person just like you, who has thoughts, feelings, worries, and concerns. Every patient is different and every case is unique, but both the patient and his or her family need to feel a sense of trust from you, and that you are taking care of them and not just treating their symptoms.

When you leave the hospital to go home, it is okay to disengage from the experiences of that day. With a metaphorical flick of the switch, find your happy place. After a long shift, go for a run, do yoga, read a book, meditate, watch TV, go fishing, play golf, write in a journal, or pursue whatever hobby you enjoy that brings you peace of mind. When you do this, you are recharging your mind, body, and spirit for the next day. It is equally therapeutic and rejuvenating.

The most important factor is that you disconnect from the experiences at the end of the shift, not before you actually walk into the patient's room.

* * *

Each part of this book has been building upon the various experiences that my parents and I went through during the summer of 2004. Every chapter has been touching upon related themes of care, communication, and compassion. The most important advice in this book, which encompasses everything that has been discussed, is this: when you walk into the patient's room, first, treat the body, and second, heal the person.

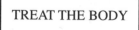

TREAT THE BODY ➡ HEAL THE PERSON

When you are working with a patient, the health status is always the top priority. You do everything in your knowledge to give them the proper medical treatment. After everything is medically attended to, then it is time to heal the person—the individual—by showing empathy, compassion, and an understanding of what he or she is going through. By addressing both sides of the spectrum, you are making a positive impact and helping to improve the overall patient experience.

Suggestions for Health Care Providers and/or Patient's Family:

- Life and death is the cycle of life. The key is not to fix your mind on the concept of dying, but on making the most of and for the living.
- People handle sadness, grief, and loss in different ways. If you have to address a difficult topic or present bad news to the patient and his or her family, they may lash out at the reality of the moment and situation, not at you personally.
- If you feel that working twelve-hour shifts is taking a mental and physical toll on your body, pursue the option of working an eight-hour shift if that is available in your department.
- Some educational programs can help mitigate burnout symptoms, improve job satisfaction, and possibly decrease the high turnover rate for ICU nurses (Mealer et al., 2012). Research programs that may be available to you.
- Treat the body, then heal the person.

Reflective Questions for Health Care Providers (write your answers in Part Five):

1) How do you consider your level of satisfaction with your career?
2) Can you list a specific time when you started to feel frustrated with your work? What helped get you through that experience?

3) What are things that you do that help you unwind after a stressful shift?

4) Based on the conversations you have with your coworkers, do you sense that feeling burned out is common in the hospital? What are the main causes of this (e.g., sick patients, administration, feeling overworked, lack of equipment, lack of support from coworkers)? Please explain.

5) What types of things do you think can be done in the workplace that will help improve the level of overall satisfaction?

PART FIVE

WORKBOOK

"I shall pass through this world but once. Any good, therefore, that I can do, or any kindness that I can show to any human being, let me do it now. Let me not defer or neglect it, for I shall not pass this way again."

—Anonymous Proverb

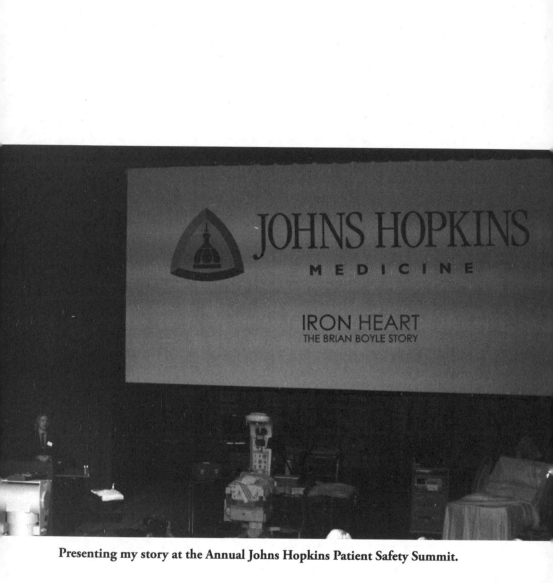

Presenting my story at the Annual Johns Hopkins Patient Safety Summit.

CHAPTER 17

A REVIEW OF SUGGESTIONS AND REFLECTIVE QUESTIONS

THIS CHAPTER IS A CONVENIENT REVIEW OF THE SUGGESTIONS AND reflective questions for health care providers that can be found in the book to provide easy access to the information; this is the appropriate place to write your answers to the reflective questions that are found at the end of each chapter.

Part One: From Tragedy to Triumph

Chapter 1: July 6, 2004

Suggestions for Health Care Providers and/or Patient's Family:

- Before you interact with patients in a situation similar to Brian's, reflect on how you could help ease the pain of a suffering family as they work through the initial shock.
- Always treat the patient as a person and not just as an injured body.
- The family wants answers on the patient's condition, and although you sometimes cannot give any answers, you can take the time to address their concerns.

Reflective Questions for Health Care Providers:

1) How often do you reflect on the patient's experience? The family's experience?

_____

_____

2) Imagine being in Brian's shoes when he started to regain consciousness. How would you feel?

_____

_____

3) Imagine the feeling that Brian's parents had when they received the phone call that Brian was in critical condition, and the feeling they had when they saw him in the recovery room for the first time. What thoughts would be going through your mind at this point in time?

_____

_____

4) Imagine being one of Brian's care providers when he first arrived at the hospital. What is one particular thing that you could do to help his loved ones adjust to the shock of the situation?

_____

_____

5) As a care provider, how do you personally find hope in a seemingly hopeless situation (i.e., stepping back from the "Oh wow, they are really sick" moment to take the appropriate steps to treat the patient)?

_____

_____

Chapter 2: A Voice for the Voiceless

Suggestions for Health Care Providers and/or Patient's Family:

- Help keep your patients focused on the positive things that they have going for them (they are alive, people believe in them, you are supporting them, etc.).
- Help keep the family members focused on the positive aspects of the patient's recovery process.
- Approach any conversation with a family member in a manner that helps put him or her at ease, as difficult as this may be sometimes. Even the tone of a voice can be significant.
- Showing sincerity and empathy goes a long way with the patient and his or her family.

Reflective Questions for Health Care Providers:

1) How would you feel if you were no longer able to physically complete the activities of daily living?

_____

_____

2) How do you physically and mentally prepare a patient and family to transition from acute care to rehabilitation?

_____

_____

3) When a patient is very focused on the negative aspects of his or her situation, how can you help him or her focus on finding the strength to keep striving toward making improvements?

_____

_____

4) After you discharge a patient, do you wonder how he or she is
    doing as he or she navigates through the health care system and
    recovery process?

    _____

    _____

5) How often do you hear how your patients are doing after they
    have been discharged? How does it make you feel knowing that
    you contributed to their recovery?

    _____

    _____

Chapter 3: Brian's Website

Suggestions for Health Care Providers and/or Patient's Family:

- The health care providers see families that are dealing with grief on
  a daily basis, but a new family that is just entering the hospital with
  their loved one has no idea what to expect. These families are often
  put in positions where they have to continuously report the patient's
  health status to every friend and family member who comes to visit
  or calls on the phone. Not every patient will be fortunate enough
  to have a lot of people coming to visit. It is heartwarming to see
  such an outpouring of generous support, but having to repeat the
  information over and over can take a heavy toll on the mind and
  body. The care provider can recommend a strategy, like providing
  daily health status updates on a website, so they do not have to
  keep repeating the same traumatic information.
- Since technology is advancing by the minute, there are a lot of
  new electronic communication sites that exist today. The hospital

could provide informational links to families or friends on how to establish a site to report their loved one's condition. The hospital could even include these details on its own website and the care providers could suggest to loved ones that they go there to find details on what websites they can choose from.

- In most cases, the people closest to the patient (parents, husband, wife, significant other, etc.) have an incredible workload just trying to take care of the patient. It might be helpful for the care provider to help the family designate a spokesperson to share news and updates on the status of the patient (via text message, phone calls, emails, and a website) so those closest to the patient will not have to worry about trying to keep others informed.

- There are many benefits to maintaining a website, especially one that has a format where people can write messages and thoughtful notes of inspiration. These encouraging messages not only help motivate everyone who has permission to view the website, but also bring strength to the closest members of the family who are looking after the patient every day. These messages can have a very motivational influence on the patient when, and if, he or she is able to view them.

Reflective Questions for Health Care Providers:

1) Do you personally believe that keeping a daily health status website can be beneficial for the patient's family? Under what circumstances? Explain why you feel that way.

_____

_____

2) When you know that a patient is going to be long term, do you recommend to his or her family that it might be helpful for them to look into creating a website that will give a daily update on the patient's health status?

_____

_____

3) If you do recommend a website to the family that will provide daily health updates, which one do you recommend the most? Why?

_____

_____

4) Can you remember a specific time that you heard about the benefits of using the website?

_____

_____

5) How should hospital personnel relate the news of an accident on the phone? How can the patient's serious condition be relayed without causing too much alarm or stress?

_____

_____

Part Two: Care

Chapter 4: Patient- and Family-Centered Care

Suggestions for Health Care Providers and/or Patient's Family:

- If there is no support group, perhaps a Point of Contact could be available for information or questions. Doctors and nurses are extremely busy and not always available.

- A hospital information guide for visitors (Appendix) would be helpful. This guide would provide hospital phone numbers, visiting hours, parking and cafeteria information, nearby hotel listings, and simple medical-term definitions. It would also be helpful to include details on what family members should expect or be required to do, including behavior. My parents saw so many rude families that had loved ones inside the unit treating the medical people badly, even to the point of trashing the waiting room. Everyone reacts to grief differently, but to take it out on the doctors and nurses trying to save lives is just not right.

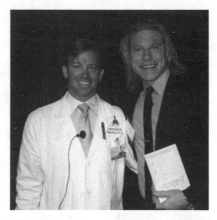

Dr. Peter Pronovost is a world-renowned leader in patient safety. I am thankful for the opportunity to collaborate with him and his team at the Armstrong Institute for Patient Safety and Quality on "Project Emerge," a revolutionary tool to help improve the level of communication among patients, families, and their health care providers.

- Listen to the feedback from the people who know the patient best (parents, family, significant others, and close friends) because they may notice a small lifesaving detail in the patient that the care providers are unable to see.

Reflective Questions for Health Care Providers:

1) Do you feel that you always try to engage with the patient? Please explain in more detail.

_____

_____

2) Do you feel that you always try to engage with the patient's family? Please explain in more detail.

_____

_____

3) Are there any circumstances that would keep you from engaging with a patient or the patient's family?

_____

_____

4) When you have a new patient and you meet his or her family for the first time, are there certain things that you do that help put them at ease?

_____

_____

5) Do you listen and engage with the patient's family and close friends to help the way that you treat the patient?

_____

_____

Chapter 5: Sensation and Perception

Suggestions for Health Care Providers and/or Patient's Family:

- If there is a TV available in the room, keep it tuned to a station that you think the patient would like. Even if the volume is turned down, just having something visual patients can look at helps increase mental stimulation.
- Music soothes the soul. Even in dire situations, like a coma, hospitals could allow families to provide a patient's favorite music,

within reason, as background noise, as long as it does not inter-fere with the medical equipment or the nurses' and doctors' work.

- If in doubt about the type of music to play for your loved one, classical music has been proven to bring about the most benefits for the patient, especially if he or she has anxiety, depressive syndromes, or are in pain or stressed (Trappe, 2010).

- If the care providers give permission, and if space is available in the patient's room, friends and family can post their letters and get well cards in an appropriate area.

- Family and friends can bring in photos they think the patient would like to see. It is a great way of bringing the patient's background into his or her new realm, because it can provide a sense of reassurance and hope that he or she can get life back to the way it was.

- When you bring in gifts for the patient, focus on bringing a token of encouragement that can be left in his or her room and seen by the patient and his or her visitors. Smaller items are better, because they will not take up too much room; think quality, not quantity.

- Turn the lights down to a lower intensity throughout the night to help improve the sleep pattern of the patient.

Reflective Questions for Health Care Providers:

1) When you are taking care of the patient, how often are you reflecting on what he or she can possibly see, hear, and feel? What are some ways that you can help improve on this?

_____

_____

2) If there are TVs or radios available in the patient's room, do you prefer to keep them turned on or off? Can you describe a specific time when you saw a patient respond to his or her surroundings in a positive way when the TV or radio was turned on?

   _____

   _____

3) If you are working with patients who are long term or unable to drink fluids for a medical reason, how often do you proceed with measures related to mouth care?

   _____

   _____

4) If family and friends have brought in photos, get well cards, and other motivational items for the patient, do you ever find yourself looking at these items to get to know your patient better? Or, do you feel that viewing these items creates too much of a personal connection with the patient?

   _____

   _____

5) What are some specific ways that you help improve the patient's atmosphere to make it personal and relaxing for him or her?

   _____

   _____

Chapter 6: Setting Goals for the Patient

Suggestions for Health Care Providers and/or Patient's Family:

•   Set realistic goals for the patient.

- Review the medical transfer file and consult with a doctor for any concerns.
- Monitor your patient closely—especially his or her heart rate, respiratory rate, breathing pattern, temperature, and blood pressure.
- Do not put the patient in a situation where the patient could get injured.
- Reflect on your progress and improvements each week.
- Alter your plans accordingly if you see that the patient is well ahead or well behind the planned schedule.

Reflective Questions for Health Care Providers:

1) When you select a long-term goal for the patient, what are the steps that you take in order to help the patient achieve it? (E.g., do you break the long-term goal into smaller goals, do you focus only on the main goal, or do you have a long-term goal in mind but keep it only to yourself without letting the patient know about it?)

_____

_____

2) Think back on a specific time when a patient of yours was getting discouraged. What did you do or say to him or her to help cheer him or her up?

_____

_____

3) If you were the patient, what types of things would inspire you to accomplish your goals?

_____

_____

4) If you were the patient, what types of things would make you feel overwhelmed or pessimistic about achieving the stated goals?

_____

_____

5) If your patient is struggling to achieve goals, what is one way that you can encourage him or her to stay positive?

_____

_____

Part Three: Communication

Chapter 7: Before Stepping into the Patient's Room

Suggestions for Health Care Providers and/or Patient's Family:

- Every time you leave one room and enter another room, it is important to reground your thoughts.
- Focus on the greater good of caring for your patient.
- When you are having a chaotic day, think about a happy memory, sing a favorite song in your head, or do something that you know will distract your mind.

Reflective Questions for Health Care Providers:

1) When you are having a hectic day, what are some of the strategies that have helped you redirect your focus and energy?

_____

_____

2) What can you do to prepare yourself before walking into a patient's room?

_____

_____

3) After being given your report/sign-out on a patient with a family that has a reputation for being difficult, how can you prepare yourself to walk into that room with an unbiased opinion?

_____

_____

4) If you are having a bad day in your personal life, what can you do to compartmentalize your feelings in order to give completely dedicated care to your patient?

_____

_____

5) If you notice a coworker is having a stressful day through his or her words or actions, what can you do to help him or her make the appropriate change in his or her attitude and behavior?

_____

_____

Chapter 8: Bedside Manners Are as Simple as a Smile

Suggestions for Health Care Providers and/or Patient's Family:

- Think about the impact you are making in the lives of your patients and their families.
- Be positive and optimistic around your patients and their families.
- Do not be afraid to talk to your patients.
- Always be aware of the importance of bedside manners when you engage with a patient and his or her family.

Reflective Questions for Health Care Providers:

1) How would you rate your bedside manners?

   _____

   _____

2) What is one recommendation that you can give to brand-new care providers on how to initiate a conversation with a patient?

   _____

   _____

3) How can you personally convey to the patient that he or she is not just a body being treated, but a person?

   _____

   _____

4) When you walk into the room of a new patient, is there a certain protocol (e.g., smile, shake hands, address by first name, sit down next to him or her) that you follow in order to make the patient feel comfortable in your presence?

   _____

   _____

5) If you were the patient, what is something that your care provider could do to make you feel at ease?

   _____

   _____

Chapter 9: Talking to the Patient and His or Her Family

Suggestions for Health Care Providers and/or Patient's Family:

- Extending ICU visiting hours could be a target for review, depending on the condition of the patient.

- Allow a family to meet the night nurse during a specified time.

- It would be helpful if there were a hospital computer system where a family representative could check medical information and the status of a patient.

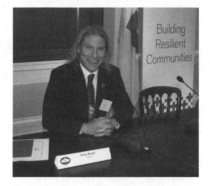

At the White House, receiving the Champion of Change award from the President of the United States of America in recognition of my Red Cross volunteer work and health care advocacy.

- Have someone to guide patients when arriving at a rehab facility. Have the person or team of people working with a patient discuss his or her medical condition, prescriptions, and rehabilitation plan so they are all on the same page when communicating with family members.

- Similar to patient and family engagement in the hospital setting, the family members could add valuable pieces of information regarding the patient in rehab.

- When you are in the patient's room, whether you know it or not, you are already interacting with him or her. A single word does not have to be spoken for an interaction to occur, but audible conversation does have a profound impact on the thoughts and feelings of the patient.

- Helping a family feel accepted by the hospital staff can be initiated by making eye contact, talking with the family, and listening to their questions (Browning & Warren, 2006).

- Have a printout or computer log the patient's family can reference, even in emergency or ICU situations, to help them understand what is going on. Some people may find it helpful to view the medical records during their hospital stay, and it may help the healing process along.

Reflective Questions for Health Care Providers:

1) When you first started working as a care provider, how did you feel the first time you interacted with the patient and his or her family? How do you feel now when you talk to them? If there has been a change over the years, why do you think this is?

   _____

   _____

2) When you witness a visitor interact with the patient, what are the signs that the patient enjoys or dislikes the presence of the visitor?

   _____

   _____

3) What are your favorite topics that you enjoy discussing with your patients and their families?

   _____

   _____

4) Is there any particular method of communication that you feel works well with patients and their families? What methods tend not to work?

_____

_____

5) What is one particular thing that you can start doing right away to improve your communication with your patients and families?

_____

_____

Chapter 10: Keeping a Journal

Suggestions for Health Care Providers and/or Patient's Family:

- Encourage the patient to keep a journal to track physical, emotional, and psychological progress and write down things that he or she may have a difficult time talking about.

- You do not have to be a patient to keep a journal. It is very effective for a family member or friend of somebody who is going through the recovery process. It is also effective for a care provider to keep a journal in order to reflect on certain patients, your interactions with them, and the overall outcomes of the people that you treat.

- The style of the journal is completely up to the writer. Do not worry about punctuation, grammar, or vocabulary. The focus is not on how the entries are written, but on what is written.

- It can be helpful to include inspirational notes throughout journal entries. These short reminders can provide added motivation that will stand out to you as you skim through the pages of the journal.

Reflective Questions for Health Care Providers:

1) What are some measures that you have your patients take in order to help them heal emotionally and psychologically? What about some measures for their families?

   _____

   _____

2) What are measures that you take to buoy your psychological and emotional well-being? Have you ever kept a journal for yourself? Why or why not?

   _____

   _____

3) Have you ever recommended to your patients that they keep a journal to document what they are thinking and feeling as they go through the recovery process? Please explain in detail.

   _____

   _____

4) Can you list a particular time when you saw or heard about one of your patients benefitting from keeping a journal?

   _____

   _____

5) If the patient is unable to write, what is an alternative method that you can suggest that might have similar benefits?

   _____

   _____

Chapter 11: Art Therapy

Suggestions for Health Care Providers and/or Patient's Family:

- Art is a very personal form of self-expression; I suggest the best place to start is with a blank canvas.

- After you start drawing a line or a shape, react to it. How does it make you feel? What does it remind you of? Let your mind roam and wander through your past, present, and future. Visually explore your hopes, fears, dreams, nightmares, worries, goals, and concerns.

- Choose whatever medium you have an interest in: drawing, painting, sculpture, photography, digital video, etc.

- Always keep in mind that this is your work of art, and you are free to create anything you would like. If you like the color blue, add as much blue in the piece as you like. If you like portraits, draw a portrait. If you prefer an Impressionist approach over more of an Abstract method, by all means, go for it.

- Remember that there are no rules or restrictions when it comes to your work. If you want to add a detail or take it out, this is completely up to you.

- The focus should be more on expression than perfection. Go with your instincts and base your decisions on how you are reacting to your art.

Reflective Questions for Health Care Providers:

1) Do you personally feel that art therapy is effective? Please explain in detail.

_____

_____

2) If you do feel that art therapy is effective, do you recommend it to your patients who you think could benefit from it? Why?

_____

_____

3) Can you list a particular time when you saw one of your patients benefit from using art as a part of his or her therapy?

_____

_____

4) Outside of writing in a journal, talking about their experiences, and using art therapy, what other measures do you think patients can take in order to help them cope with the stress they are going through?

_____

_____

5) What types of factors in patients' behavior and outlook would you look for when thinking about incorporating art therapy into their treatment plan?

_____

_____

Part Four: Compassion

Chapter 12: Seeing the World Through the Eyes of the Patient

Suggestions for Health Care Providers and/or Patient's Family:

- Try to keep negative stimuli from patients and their families. Remember that visitors are most likely inexperienced and unacquainted with the hospital environment, and the sights and scenes may be alarming to them.

- Try to always be sensitive to the tremendous "battles" patients and their families have fought and will fight in the future.

Reflective Questions for Health Care Providers:

1) How can you become engaged with your coworkers, patients, and visitors? What are some simple ways you can show people you care?

_____

_____

2) How can you show your commitment to your organization's vision and mission? Do you think your level of commitment will trickle down to your patient care strategy?

_____

_____

3) Try to remember a time when you experienced a small triumph with a patient as he or she accomplished a goal. How did this make you feel?

_____

_____

4) Do you think that having your patients and their families see other patients and their families in similar situations will help them heal and cope? How so?

_____

_____

5) How do you deal with the unfairness (e.g., who lives and who dies) of life and how precarious life can be?

_____

_____

Chapter 13: The Golden Rule

Suggestions for Health Care Providers and/or Patient's Family:

- Speak in a gentle tone of voice. Use the family's names and the name of the patient frequently; this shows them that you are acknowledging their family and their loved one.
- Use uplifting words and phrases as often as possible because they will create a positive atmosphere.
- Try to form a connection with patients and families to establish a sense of trust before you give them any medical updates.
- Reflect on the type of family you are talking to, and present the information in a compassionate way rather than just stating the facts.
- Provide realistic expectations that they should have regarding treatment and progress.

Reflective Questions for Health Care Providers:

1) If you were the family member, what would you like to hear in order to help alleviate pain as the reality of the situation sets in? What are things that you would not like to hear?

_____

_____

2) In your experiences as a care provider, what are specific measures that you have taken to connect with a patient and his or her

family? Which measures worked best, and which measures did not work at all?

_____

_____

3) What can you say to the family about what you are doing for the patient without giving false promises? (E.g., "We are doing all that we can, but we have to wait and see.")

_____

_____

4) How can you encourage your patient to realize that even small goals matter?

_____

_____

5) How can you encourage the family of the patient to appreciate that even small improvements are monumental events taking place?

_____

_____

Chapter 14: The Stages of Grief

Suggestions for Health Care Providers and/or Patient's Family:

- When dealing with the grief of the patient and his or her family, offer reassurance and support.
- Try to remember and recognize all the stages of grief.
- Remember not to take things personally when a family is distraught.

- As a care provider, remember that you are the biggest ally for the family and that you have the power to help guide them through the recovery process, both the ups and the downs.

Reflective Questions for Health Care Providers:

1) How did you feel the first time you observed a patient's loved ones going through the various stages of grief? How do you feel now when you see it?

   _____

   _____

2) How do you prepare yourself before you have to give bad news to a patient or a patient's family member?

   _____

   _____

3) When you do have to present bad news to a patient or family, do you feel that you disconnect from the situation to help get you through the conversation? What helps you mentally recover after you give bad news?

   _____

   _____

4) Is there anything you have noticed over the years that has helped the family reach a sense of closure?

   _____

   _____

5) What is a measure that you take with the patient's loved ones when they refuse to accept bad news and take the frustration out on you? Please explain.

_____

_____

Chapter 15: Why Do Some Patients Heal, while Others Do Not?

Suggestions for Health Care Providers and/or Patient's Family:

- Do not take a single second for granted.
- Take the time out of your day to tell those close to you that you love them.
- Smile more and frown less.
- Show gratitude.
- Perform random acts of kindness for friends and strangers.
- Do not hold grudges.
- Be thankful for what you have and the problems that you do not have.

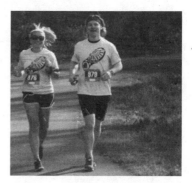

Running with my wife, Pamela, at my Iron Heart 5K, a race dedicated to health care providers. Pam is a pediatric nurse practitioner and she inspires me every day.

- Volunteer for a cause that you believe in.
- Get out of your comfort zone every once in a while and try something new.
- Be positive and optimistic.
- Go for a long walk to breathe in the life all around you.
- Make every step, every heartbeat, every moment, and every day count.

Reflective Questions for Health Care Providers:

1) What are three things that you can do today to show somebody in your life that you think he or she is special?

    _____

    _____

2) Identify a time when you can recall feeling down and another person helped you.

    _____

    _____

3) Who inspires and motivates you? Why?

    _____

    _____

4) How does the work that you do help contribute to making society a better place?

    _____

    _____

5) Can you think of possible ways to encourage patients who seem to have lost their motivation? List some.

    _____

    _____

Chapter 16: Avoiding Burnout Syndrome

Suggestions for Health Care Providers and/or Patient's Family:

- Life and death is the cycle of life. The key is not to fix your mind on the concept of dying, but on making the most of and for the living.

- People handle sadness, grief, and loss in different ways. If you have to address a difficult topic or present bad news to the patient and his or her family, they may lash out at the reality of the moment and situation, not at you personally.

- If you feel that working twelve-hour shifts is taking a mental and physical toll on your body, pursue the option of working an eight-hour shift if that is available in your department.

- Some educational programs can help mitigate burnout symptoms, improve job satisfaction, and possibly decrease the high turnover rate for ICU nurses (Mealer et al., 2012). Research programs that may be available to you.

- Treat the body, then heal the person.

Reflective Questions for Health Care Providers:

1) How do you consider your level of satisfaction with your career?

_____

_____

2) Can you list a specific time when you started to feel frustrated with your work? What helped get you through that experience?

_____

_____

3) What are things that you do that help you unwind after a stressful shift?

_____

_____

4) Based on the conversations you have with your coworkers, do you sense that feeling burned out is common in the hospital?

What are the main causes of this (e.g., sick patients, administration, feeling overworked, lack of equipment, lack of support from coworkers)? Please explain.

_____

_____

5) What types of things do you think can be done in the workplace that will help improve the level of overall satisfaction?

_____

_____

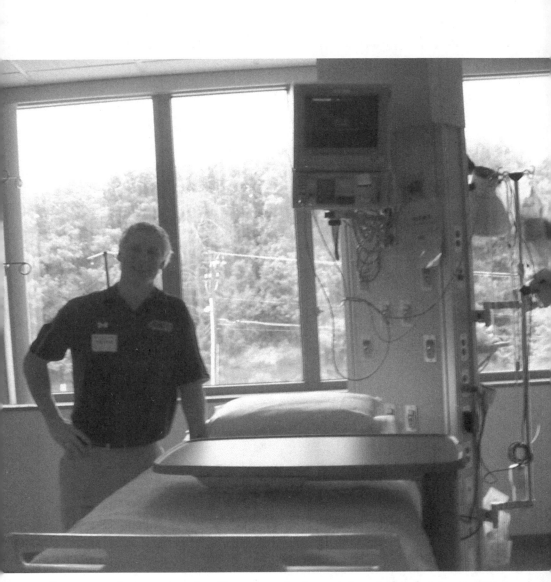

It was very therapeutic to be able to come back to my hospital and visit room 19 in the ICU.

CHAPTER 18

SIMULATION EXERCISES TO IMPROVE THE PATIENT EXPERIENCE

W E COULD DISCUSS THE PATIENT EXPERIENCE AND THE IMPORTANCE OF bedside manners in full detail for another thousand pages and it still would not do this topic enough justice. There is more than reading about being aware of the patient and his or her family to learning exactly what to do when we walk into the patient's room.

When it comes to mastering the patient experience, we must pursue it like every other skill—by studying, preparing, practicing, applying, and then perfecting it over time. These exercises will help apply the information that we have been discussing in real-world scenarios.

Exercise 1—Observe, Reflect, React

AS A CARE PROVIDER, WHEN YOU WALK INTO THE PATIENT'S ROOM, YOU *observe* the patient's condition by checking his or her vital signs, blood pressure, IV fluids, medication, respiration rate, level of comfort, etc. As you process this information, you *reflect* on the next step that you need to do for the patient, and then you *react* by doing it.

These three measures are important when it comes to medically treating the patient, but they are also influential when it comes to emotionally treating the patient and his or her family. In the same way that you walk into the patient's room and observe his or her physical functions and symptoms, you also *observe* the patient's emotional stability (e.g., sensation and stimulation engagement, communication, conversation, comfort with external environment). You *reflect* on how you can make his or her external environment more comfortable for the patient, and then *react* by doing it.

In this exercise, we are going to look at a few scenarios that will help us see life through the eyes of the patient and family so that we can be aware of their world and do what we can to improve it.

1) As a care provider, you walk into the patient's room. The patient is male, middle-aged, semi-conscious, recovering from heart surgery, and visibly showing his awareness by making subtle attempts to respond to your commands after being unconscious for the past seven days. He tends to get easily agitated. He has not received any visits from family or friends. What can you say to him to provide comfort? Is there anything that you can do to improve his level of comfort? Please explain.

_____

_____

A. If you were the patient, what type of things would you like the care provider to do to tend to your emotional needs and sensory perception? Please explain.

_____

_____

2) As a care provider, you walk into the patient's room. The patient is female, teenaged, and has been medically induced into a coma

for fourteen days after a very serious car accident. Her ability to respond to commands is subtle, and she is showing an improvement in her levels of awareness as she is being weaned off sedation. Her parents and brother are at her bedside during each session of visiting hours. Do you talk to her? What do you say? What can you do to make sure her environment is as comfortable as possible? What measures can you take to improve her mental stimulation and help tend to her senses? Please explain.

_____

_____

A.   As the care provider, what can you do to engage with her parents? While keeping the expectations realistic, how can you help put them at ease and provide comfort when appropriate?

_____

_____

B.   If you were the patient, what type of things would you like the care provider to do to help tend to your emotional needs and sensory perception? Please explain.

_____

_____

C.   If you were her parents, what type of things would you like the care provider to do in order to help you feel at ease? Please explain.

_____

_____

Exercise 2—Patient Care Diagram

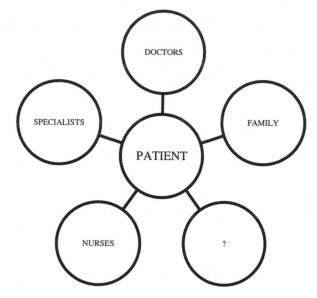

Patient Care Diagram

IN THE DIAGRAM, THE PATIENT IS AT THE CENTER. AROUND THE RADIAL are four groups that work together to help the patient through the recovery process. These groups include

Family: Parents, guardians, relatives, significant others, and close friends

Doctors: Physicians, surgeons, nurse practitioners, physician assistants, radiologists, psychiatrists, and psychologists

Nurses: Expertise is based on the department of the hospital that they work in

Specialists: Respiratory therapists, occupational therapists, physical therapists, speech and language pathologists, nutritionists, case managers, and social workers

* Disclaimer: There are many disciplines and titles in the field of health care. In this example I have chosen to use the backgrounds of my care providers in order to simplify the concept. If your discipline or professional area is not listed, I have organized these categories so it will be easy for you to choose the category that you fit in.

In the blank circle, identify another group that you feel contributes to the care plan of the patient. Explain that group's role.

_____

_____

From your experience, do you feel that any of these groups have more of an influence on the type of care plan that is created for the patient? Why do you feel that way?

_____

_____

From your experience, who do you think knows the patient best out of these groups?

_____

_____

The aim of this exercise is not to see who has the most power and influence regarding the treatment of the patient, but to have a discussion about how each of these groups contributes to the patient's observation and type of treatment. Why is it important to have all these groups working together when it comes to caring for the patient? Please explain.

_____

_____

Exercise 3—Through the Eyes of the Patient

This final exercise will help you tap into the mindset of a patient who is aware, yet unable to communicate. The ideal location to conduct this exercise is in a simulation lab, with real sounds from medical equipment to replicate the environment of a hospital room. However, the exercise can also be done alone in your home.

To begin the exercise, lie on a relatively flat surface such as a bed, a couch, or even a carpeted floor. Lie still for twenty minutes without talking or moving any part of your body. The only thing that you can move is your eyes.

1) As you lay there, what type of thoughts were going through your mind? Please explain.

   _____

   _____

2) How did your body feel? Were you comfortable? Please explain.

   _____

   _____

3) First, were you able to stay in the position for the entire twenty minutes without moving? How many more minutes do you think you could have stayed in this position? Explain.

   _____

   _____

The goal of this exercise is to briefly simulate the patient experience. I congratulate you if you were able to reach the goal by staying perfectly still for the entire twenty minutes. Do you think you could have done it if your senses were continuously bombarded with beeping and buzzing from the medical equipment next to your hospital bed? Or seeing your family and friends come into your room and hysterically beg you to stay strong? Or having tubes and wires running through your body? Or overhearing conversations of how your health is failing and, at any minute, they would be transferring you to a nursing home for long-term care?

The patient is not simulating this exercise for twenty minutes; he or she is experiencing this arduous reality for hours, days, and even weeks. Not only that, but based on the patient's circumstances, his or her life could be hanging by a single thread, which heightens the intensity. It is practically impossible to comprehend all of this without being a patient, but the more you try, the easier it becomes for you to understand what the patient is going through. The more you can understand the patient's experience, the more you can help improve his or her quality of life while confined to a hospital bed.

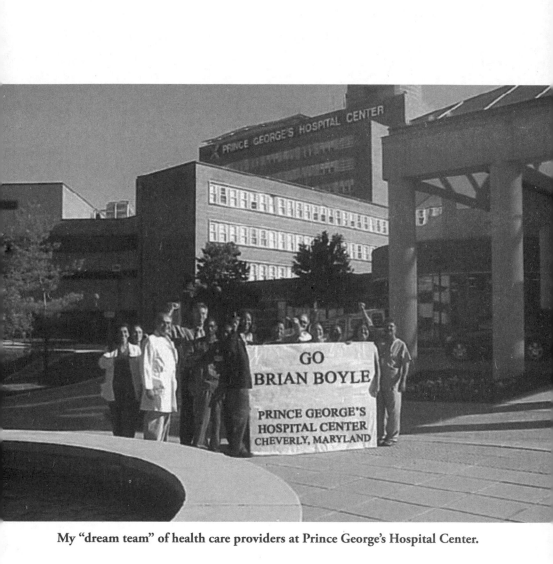

My "dream team" of health care providers at Prince George's Hospital Center.

EPILOGUE:
A MESSAGE OF APPRECIATION
TO HEALTH CARE PROVIDERS

We turn on the radio on our way to work and we are inundated with tragic news about the murders that have occurred overnight in some part of the city, the natural disasters that are tearing up the land in some part of the country, and the warfare that is spreading like an incurable disease in some part of the world—not to mention the medical crisis occurring in our world today. As a society, we have become so used to witnessing sadness and devastation on a grand scale. More often than not, we see the hardship and downfall of the human spirit across our news feeds and television stations. But, what about the triumph of the human spirit? Like a tiny diamond surrounded by dense rock, there are ordinary people who are accomplishing extraordinary things that are helping our world become a better place.

At this very minute, in hospitals all over the world, there are people who are treating the sick, wounded, and dying. These people not only are saving individuals, but are breathing life back into families and supporting causes that they believe will make a positive difference in their communities. Just like the brave men and women who serve in our nation's military and the people who protect our everyday safety and freedom, health care providers and EMS professionals protect our lives and are included in this group that makes our world work, and thrive, and live. The people who walk into work, light up a room, and make things happen.

As a former ICU patient, I not only represent the result of the life-saving capabilities of modern medicine, but also represent the hard work of my care providers. I am eternally thankful for the gift of life that they have given me, and the life that all care providers provide their patients.

I know that working in the field of health care can be a challenge, because there are goals that have to be reached and things that have to be financially managed and accounted for. When we step back to look at the big picture, we see that the work being done does not just change numbers; it affects people. These people have backgrounds, they have families, and they have lives. That body in the hospital bed is a person, and it is so important to remember this when the numbers and different financial goals are being discussed in the media. You do not get the credit you truly deserve because what you are doing is saving these people, saving their hopes for the future, saving families, and saving communities. This is the result of your hard work, your expertise, and your dedication to what you do.

I know that I am not a doctor, nurse, physical therapist, or hospital administrator. However, my knowledge is based on personal experience. I do not have a medical degree or a nursing license, but I do have memories that I am reminded of every time I see my scars in a mirror. I never forget that I almost died during the summer of 2004, so these memories are constant reminders that I am alive because of these people. I was given the privilege of looking back, which is a major reason for writing this second book.

I have talked about the experiences that my parents and I went through in great detail in the previous chapters, referring to certain moments of my treatment that really stood out to us, and offering suggestions where we thought they were necessary. I had a great team of care providers, and I am eternally grateful for everything they did for me while I was a patient. These hardworking individuals whom I saw every day became my friends and an extended family. These people watched over me every day and helped alleviate my suffering while I lay there in what was almost my deathbed.

After spending over two months in the ICU, I felt that I knew more about room 19 than my own bedroom in my house. There was a connection there that I cannot quite explain. I could tell you every specific and exact object that was in that room. The off-white walls, the checkered floor with pinkish tiles, the aqua-colored chair to the right of me by the fan, the sink and table on the left side of the room, the bulletin board on the left wall, and the clock above the doorway. I can tell you which nurses and doctors worked on what shifts, and what type of food would be served at each time of day.

My hospital room was my sanctuary, a temporary safe haven from surgery and agony. I felt that I was free of pain when I was in my hospital bed, and the moment I was wheeled outside of my room, I knew that I would be going somewhere unpleasant. I knew that I would be having tests done on my heart, lungs, kidneys, liver, brain, and other vital organs—tests that took up a majority of my time there. If I was not going to get a test done, then I would most likely be going to the operating room to get ripped open again.

I was very sad when the time came for me to be transferred to the step-down unit to prepare for my new life full of rehab as I learned to regain my independence. I did not want to leave the ICU, as I had become so used to being there that I did not think I could handle being anywhere else. What would my life be like outside of that room? I forgot what the world was like outside of the hospital, because room 19 had become my entire universe.

Home really is where the heart is, and room 19 in the ICU was my second home. I did not want to leave my nurses, therapists, and doctors—my friends. They watched over me like guardian angels, waiting and hoping for my recovery to progress. With every second that ticked by, they patiently waited to give me a helping hand back into life. There was a bond that was made with these people that only grew stronger the more I progressed. It was the same feeling that you have when you are standing around your close friends at your high school graduation ceremony, knowing that you will soon be going on separate paths and probably will not see a lot of these people for a long time or ever again. Deep in my heart, the heart that they helped mend over and over, their memories would remain with me.

You cannot understand what it is like to be a patient unless you have been a patient or have witnessed a loved one in the hospital. It is not an easy journey to take, and it is not something you can come to understand overnight. Processing the information in the previous chapters will help you gain a little better insight into the perspective of the patient.

Like I have said many times throughout these chapters, every patient has a story and an experience. My story is one of many, and my parents and I have done our best to represent these courageous individuals and their families.

By taking the time to read this book, you have embraced what it means to see the world through the eyes of the patient and his or her family. It is our hope that with this information, you can improve the patient experience in your noble health care career and always be aware of the importance of care, communication, and compassion in the hospital room.

When you work in the field of health care, you are responsible for either bringing people back to life, or making them comfortable for the rest of their lives. Yes, some days are better than others, but every day is a great day when you help others in need, especially when they depend on you not only to live, but to live a full, meaningful life as well.

In whatever part of the health care system you work, I would like to thank you for choosing this path in life, and for all that you do every day for your patients and their families.

ACKNOWLEDGMENTS

I APPROACHED THE WRITING OF THIS BOOK SIMILARLY TO HOW I PREPARE for an Ironman triathlon or a marathon. I did all the research that I possibly could and when it was time to begin writing, I focused on handling each of the elements along the way. This path may have been pursued individually, but in no way was this process an individual effort. I always give credit where it is due, and this book has been a team effort from the very beginning.

I would like to start off by thanking Alison Burrows and Mark Rulle from the Maryland Healthcare Education Institute for supporting me all these years and helping me share my story and experiences in the health care setting on a national level. I would also like to thank Carmela Coyle and the amazing team at the Maryland Hospital Association for all the encouragement with my health care advocacy, especially my friend David Simon, who provided a lot of guidance and editorial support throughout writing this book.

As the National Volunteer Spokesperson of the American Red Cross, it has been a privilege to volunteer for a cause in which I believe with all of my heart. My gratitude goes out to all my Red Cross friends across the country, including my team at the Greater Chesapeake & Potomac Blood Services Region; National Headquarters in Washington, DC; Donna Morrissey;

Jecoliah Ellis; Dr. Mary O'Neill; Kay Schwartz; Brian Hamil; Michael Kempesty; Mary Brant; Courtney Junkin; Peggy Dyer; Shaun Gilmore; Darren Irby; Linda Voss; and Steve Mavica. I believe in the role of strong leadership and a special thanks goes out to the president and CEO of the American Red Cross, Gail McGovern, for always believing in me and supporting my mission to raise awareness on the importance of blood donation.

I chose to write this book as a part of my practicum for my Master of Arts in Communications at Johns Hopkins University. My appreciation goes out to the president of the university, Ron Daniels, and to all my professors in the communications department, especially Susan Allen, who has been a guiding force with the structure, organization, and content of the book. I would also like to thank Dr. Peter Pronovost and his team at the Armstrong Institute for Patient Safety and Quality for all the motivation to continue with my mission in improving the patient experience in the hospital setting.

This book would not exist if it were not for my incredible team at Skyhorse Publishing in New York City, including Tony Lyons, Jennifer McCartney, Bill Wolfsthal, Jay Cassell, and Lindsey Breuer. I never thought I would be a published author, and I thank my friend and coauthor of *Iron Heart*, Bill Katovsky, for all that he has done to help me with my writing career.

My heart goes out to all the care providers who played a helping hand in my survival, from my EMS providers to my care providers in the hospital to everyone who helped me get back on my feet. The sincere appreciation I have for you goes beyond words. You did not just save me, you saved my family, and we are eternally grateful.

My appreciation goes out to my family and friends for always being there to support me on every step of this journey. My grandfather, Joe

Lineberger, taught me at a young age about determination and why it is so important to turn challenges into opportunities for growth. My mother-in-law, Linda Franco-DiPiazza, taught me about the compassion and dedication of being an ICU nurse; thank you for all that you have done in your nursing career spanning over two decades.

Thanks to my mom and dad for always being there for me, in sickness and in health. Your strength gave me strength in times when I desperately needed it. You were the light in my darkness. I am blessed to call you my parents, but you are also my heroes.

To my wonderful wife, Pamela, thank you for your guidance with this project, for all that you do as a pediatric nurse, and for your love. While I was on my deathbed, my dad begged me to stay strong and to keep fighting to live—for them, for myself, and for my future wife and children. I did not completely understand the magnitude of that statement until the day I married you. You are my inspiration.

SAMPLE INFORMATION PAMPHLET FOR FAMILIES

HOSPITAL INFORMATION GUIDE FOR VISITORS (Page 1 of 2)
As a visitor in the hospital, you are spending most of your time trying to attend to your loved one, the patient. Throughout this experience, it can feel like you are walking this path by yourself, but you are not alone. These are helpful suggestions, reminders, and recommendations that we have created to help take care of you, as you help take care of your loved one.
PHONE NUMBERS Main Line: Directory: Financial: Administrative/Medical Records:
HOSPITAL HOURS Cafeteria: Chapel: Parking: Security: Blood Donation Center:
VISITING HOURS Emergency Room: ICU: Cardiology: Medical/Surgical: Labor & Delivery: Mental Health:
ADMISSION RULES Allowances for patients (e.g., music, fan, food):
SAMPLE MEDICAL TERMS AND DEFINITIONS Angiogram: CAT Scan: MRI: X-Ray: Blood Transfusion: Living Will:
REHABILITATION FACILITIES Sample #1: Sample #2:
LOCAL HOTELS Sample #1: Sample #2:

HOSPITAL INFORMATION GUIDE FOR VISITORS (Page 2 of 2)

ITEMS TO BRING WITH YOU TO THE HOSPITAL

- Bring an extra change of clothes in your vehicle, along with toiletries (e.g., toothbrush, comb, deodorant, and face wash).
- Wear comfortable shoes and dress in layers, because the hospital can get chilly and having these extra layers could transform into an instant blanket or pillow.
- It is important to stay hydrated and keep your energy levels up. Carry a small bag where you can have easy access to a water bottle and a snack.
- In between visiting hour sessions, it is helpful to occupy yourself with activities to ease your mind. If you like music, bring an iPod or a personal CD player so you can play music that helps you to relax. If you like to read, bring a book, a favorite magazine, a crossword puzzle, or an electronic reading tablet.
- Bring a notepad and a pen so you can take notes and write down questions you may have.

IMPORTANT INFORMATION TO REMEMBER

- You know the patient best. If there is something that you notice that does not look right to you, please contact the care providers and address your concern immediately.
- Be mindful that your care team is doing all they can to help take care of your loved one.
- Please do not disrupt your care providers' routines and the measures they are taking to treat the patient.
- Please be courteous and respectful of the other patients and families in the hospital. The people in the next room could be receiving devastating news and saying their final good-byes.
- Please keep your speaking voice at an appropriate level.
- You are hearing a lot of advanced medical terminology. Write down the words that you are unsure of, and look up their definitions at a later time or ask one of the care providers.
- The recovery process can be a roller-coaster ride of ups and downs. It is important to stay hopeful, maintain realistic goals, and be prepared to face setbacks.
- Rest is very important for you and the patient.

NOTES

_____
_____
_____
_____
_____
_____

REFERENCES

Barnett, L., & Chambers, M. (1996). *Reiki energy medicine: Bringing healing touch into home, hospital, and hospice.* Rochester, VT: Healing Arts Press.

Briggs, T. (2011). Music's unspoken messages. *Creative Nursing, 17*(4), 184–186.

Browning, G., & Warren, N. A. (2006). Unmet needs of family members in the medical intensive care waiting room. *Critical Care Nursing Quarterly, 29*(1), 86–95.

Desai, S., Chau, T., & George, L. (2013). Intensive care unit delirium. *Critical Care Nursing Quarterly, 36*(4), 370–389.

Fan, Y., Guo, Y., Li, Q., & Zhu, X. (2012). A review: Nursing of intensive care unit delirium. *Journal of Neuroscience Nursing, 44*(6), 307–316.

Firlik, K. S. (2006). *Another day in the frontal lobe: A brain surgeon exposes life on the inside.* New York, NY: Random House.

Flach, F. (1988). *Resilience: Discovering a new strength at times of stress.* New York, NY: Fawcett Columbine.

Gawande, A. (2007). *Better: A surgeon's notes on performance.* New York, NY: Metropolitan Books.

Gaynor, M. (1999). *Sounds of healing: A physician reveals the therapeutic power of sound, voice, and music.* New York, NY: Broadway Books.

Geiger-Brown, J., Rogers, V. E., Trinkoff, A. M., Kane, R. L., Bausell, R. B., & Scharf, S. M. (2012). Sleep, sleepiness, fatigue, and performance of 12-hour-shift nurses. *Chronobiology International, 29*(2), 211–219.

Glanz, K., Rimer, B. K., & Viswanath, K. (2008). *Health behavior and health education: Theory, research, and practice.* San Francisco, California: Jossey-Bass.

Golant, M., & Golant, S. K. (2007). *What to do when someone you love is depressed: A practical, compassionate, and helpful guide.* New York, NY: Holt Paperbacks.

Institute for Patient- and Family-Centered Care website. (2010). Retrieved October 1, 2014, from http://www.ipfcc.org/faq.html

International Center for Reiki Training website. (2014). Retrieved October 1, 2014, from http://www.reiki.org/FAQ/WhatIsReiki.html

Kieft, R. A., de Brouwer, B.B., Francke, A. L., & Delnoij, D.M. (2014). How nurses and their work environment affect patient experiences of the quality of care: A qualitative study. *BMC Health Services Research, 14(*1), 118–137.

Kirshenbaum, M. (2004). *Everything happens for a reason: Finding the true meaning of the events in our lives.* New York, NY: Harmony Books.

Kübler-Ross, E. (1977). *On death and dying.* New York, NY: Scribner.

Livesay, S., Mokracek, Sebastian, S., & Hickey, J. V. (2005). Nurses' perceptions of open visiting hours in neuroscience intensive care unit. *Journal of Nursing Care Quality, 20*(2), 182–189.

Maniou, M. (2012). Delirium: A distressing and disturbing clinical event in a intensive care unit. *Health Science Journal, 6*(4), 587–597.

Mealer, M., Jones, J., Newman, J., McFann, K., Rothbaum, B., & Moss, M. (2012). The presence of resilience is associated with a healthier psychological profile in intensive care unit (ICU) nurses: Results of a national survey. *International Journal of Nursing Studies, 49*(3), 292–299.

Pekkanen, J. (1988). M.D.: *Doctor's talk about themselves.* New York, NY: Delacorte Press.

Pifalo, T. (2007). Jogging the cogs: Trauma-focused art therapy and cognitive behavioral therapy sexually abused children. *Art Therapy: Journal of the American Art Therapy Association, 24*(2), 170–175.

Pronovost, P., & Vohr, E. (2010). *Safe patients, smart hospitals: How one doctor's checklist can help us change health care from the inside out.* New York, NY: Plume.

Sacco, T. L., Stapleton, M. F., & Ingersoll, G. L. (2009). Support groups facilitated by families of former patients: Creating family-inclusive critical care units. *Critical Care Nurse, 29*(3), 36–45.

Talwar, S. (2007). Accessing traumatic memory through art making: An art therapy protocol (ATTP). *The Arts in Psychotherapy, 34*(1), 22–35.

Trappe, H. (2010). The effects of music on the cardiovascular system and cardiovascular health. *Heart, 96*(23), 1868–1871.

Trappe, H. (2012). Role of music in intensive care medicine. *International Journal of Critical Illness and Injury Science, 2*(1), 27–31.

Ubel, P. A. (2012). *Critical decisions: How you and your doctor can make the right medical choices together.* New York, NY: Harper Collins.

Van Horn, E. R., & Kautz, D. (2007). Promotion of family integrity in the acute care setting: A review of the literature. *Dimensions of Critical Care Nursing, 26*(3), 101–107.

Warren, N. (2012). Involving patient and family advisors in the patient and family-centered care model. *MEDSURG Nursing, 21*(4), 233–239.